Urodynamics, Neurourology and Pelvic Floor Dysfunctions

Series Editor
Vincenzo Li Marzi, Urology Department, AOU Careggi University Hospital, Florence, Italy

The aim of the book series is to highlight new knowledge on physiopathology, diagnosis and treatment in the fields of pelvic floor dysfunctions, incontinence and neurourology for specialists (urologists, gynecologists, neurologists, pediatricians, physiatrists), nurses, physiotherapists and institutions such as universities and hospitals.

Gianfranco Lamberti • Cosimo De Nunzio
Editors

Bladder, Bowel and Sexual Dysfunctions Rehabilitation after Radical Prostatectomy

Surgery and Rehabilitation against Disability

Springer

Editors
Gianfranco Lamberti
Department of Rehabilitation Medicine
Ausl Piacenza
Piacenza, Italy

Cosimo De Nunzio
Urology Department
Sapienza University of Rome
Rome, Italy

ISSN 2510-4047 ISSN 2510-4055 (electronic)
Urodynamics, Neurourology and Pelvic Floor Dysfunctions
ISBN 978-3-031-76340-3 ISBN 978-3-031-76341-0 (eBook)
https://doi.org/10.1007/978-3-031-76341-0

This Springer imprint is published by the registered company Springer Nature Switzerland AG
The registered company address is: Gewerbestrasse 11, 6330 Cham, Switzerland

Preface

It is my pleasure to introduce this volume, entitled *Bladder, Bowel and Sexual Dysfunctions Rehabilitation After Radical Prostatectomy: Surgery and Rehabilitation Against Disability*. There are several reasons for being honored to present this book.

First and foremost, this publication is the latest in the series *Urodynamics, Neurourology and Pelvic Floor Dysfunctions*, resulting from a collaboration between Springer and the Italian Society of Urodynamics (SIUD), which aims to address various topics in functional urology in a straightforward yet exhaustive manner.

Second, due to the current minimally invasive techniques that aim to preserve function and facilitate rehabilitation, the management of bladder, bowel, and sexual dysfunction following prostate or bladder radical surgery has become a highly relevant topic in recent times.

Another reason why I appreciate this text is the expertise of the authors who edited it. Each of them represents a high level of ability in their respective fields. The result is a well-organized text in which contributions and different points of view come together in a practical method to produce an up-to-date addition. In fact, as is common in our series, but especially in this instance, a multidisciplinary and multiprofessional approach is the cornerstone of this volume. This text will engage the interests of urologists, physicians specializing in physical medicine and rehabilitation, as well as physiotherapists and nurses.

Finally, the presentation of this volume takes place at the end of my 3-year term as President of SIUD.

I take this opportunity to thank the editors, Cosimo De Nunzio and Gianfranco Lamberti, as well as all the authors for their countless efforts.

Enjoy reading this latest valuable addition to the editorial series of Springer volumes edited by the Italian Society of Urodynamics.

Siena, Italy Vincenzo Li Marzi

Contents

1 Bladder, Bowel, and Sexual Dysfunction After Prostatectomy and Cystoprostatectomy: Anatomical and Physiopathological Considerations

Luca Orecchia, Georges Mjaess, and Simone Albisinni

1.1 Introduction

Prostate and bladder cancer represent a major health concern in developed countries [1, 2]. The surgical management of these pathologies requires extensive knowledge of the pelvic anatomy and a profound understanding of the modifications that surgical intervention will determine on key pelvic structures. Since the introduction of laparoscopy in the early 2000s [3] and given the surge of robotics [2], surgeons have been allowed to discover and understand an anatomy which was previously hidden by the deep and complex localization of the pelvis [4]. New surgical approaches have been developed in prostate surgery, thanks to robotic-assisted surgery, such as the Retzius-sparing approach [5], the lateral approach [6], and the hood technique [7]. Apart from potentially improving patient outcomes, these techniques have prompted a new understanding of the pelvic structure and physiology. Moreover,

Luca Orecchia and Georges Mjaess contributed equally with all other contributors.

L. Orecchia
Urology Unit, Department of Surgical Sciences, Policlinico Tor Vergata University Hospital, University of Rome Tor Vergata, Rome, Italy

G. Mjaess
Department of Urology, Hôpital Universitaire de Bruxelles, Université Libre de Bruxelles, Brussels, Belgium

S. Albisinni (✉)
Urology Unit, Department of Surgical Sciences, Policlinico Tor Vergata University Hospital, University of Rome Tor Vergata, Rome, Italy

Department of Urology, Hôpital Universitaire de Bruxelles, Université Libre de Bruxelles, Brussels, Belgium

G. Lamberti, C. De Nunzio (eds.), *Bladder, Bowel and Sexual Dysfunctions Rehabilitation after Radical Prostatectomy*, Urodynamics, Neurourology and Pelvic Floor Dysfunctions, https://doi.org/10.1007/978-3-031-76341-0_1

the complex neurovascular anatomy of the bladder and prostate has been extensively restudied following the deep exploration of periprostatic tissues performed during robotic-assisted prostatectomy [8].

Modern-day surgeons must study pelvic anatomy and understand the consequences of prostate and bladder surgery, in the continuous effort to improve surgical outcomes, reduce morbidity, and enhance patient recovery and quality of life after surgery. The aim of this chapter is to define and explain the anatomical and physiopathological changes induced by such surgical procedures.

1.2 Key Anatomical Landmarks of the Male Pelvis

1.2.1 The Bladder

The bladder is a preperitoneal organ functioning as the capacitive urine reservoir and is located in the anterior portion of the pelvis minor. Its boundaries are the following:

- Anteriorly: The pubis, the umbilicovesical fascia, and, when the bladder is full, the abdominal wall. The prevesical space of Retzius is a virtual space that is easily cleavable after the opening of the fascia transversalis. It contains the Santorini venous plexus and gives access laterally to the iliac vessels and the ureters.
- Posteriorly: In men, the bladder fundus is in contact with the base of the prostate, the seminal vesicles, the vas deferens, and the rectovesical pouch of Douglas behind (Fig. 1.1).
- Laterally: The pelvic floor, the endopelvic fascia, the umbilical artery, and the vas deferens in men (Fig. 1.1).

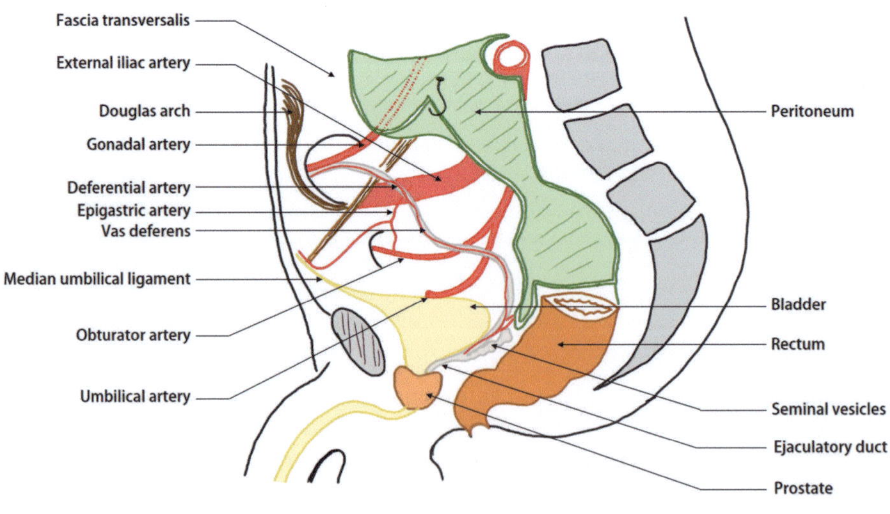

Fig. 1.1 Sagittal section of the male pelvis

The bladder is vascularized by three main arterial branches, the origin of which is the internal iliac artery. From a surgical point of view, there are lateral and posterior pedicles which, when the bladder is approached through the rectovesical space, are respectively lateral and posteromedial to the ureter. These pedicles correspond to the lateral and posterior vesical ligaments in men.

1.2.2 The Prostate

The prostate is also located in the pelvis minor, underneath the bladder. It encircles the prostatic urethra and is crossed by the ejaculatory ducts. It has a chestnut shape with an upper base, a lower apex, a lateral-ventral facet, and a dorsal facet. The striated sphincter envelops the prostatic apex and the membranous urethra. The prostate boundaries are the following (Fig. 1.2):

- Anteriorly: The retropubic space (Retzius space), the venous plexus of Santorini, and the striated urethral sphincter. The prostate also is fixed anteriorly by the puboprostatic ligaments.
- Posteriorly: The Denonvilliers's fascia and the anorectal angle.
- Laterally: The endopelvic fascia and the levator ani, separating it from the obturator foramen.

The prostate is vascularized by the inferior vesical artery (which gives rise to the vesiculodeferential arteries and vesicoprostatic arteries) and the pudendal artery.

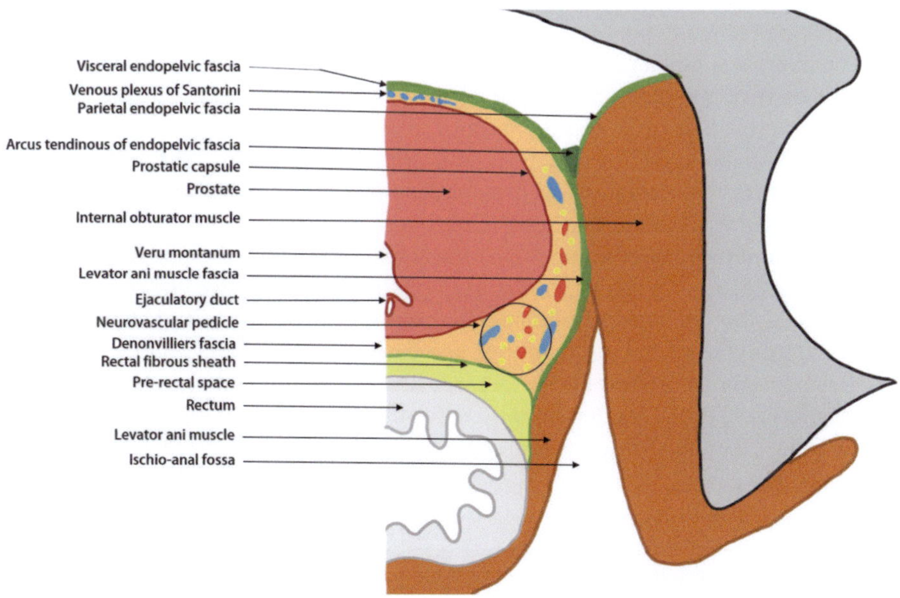

Fig. 1.2 Hemitransverse section of the male pelvis

1.2.3 Pelvic Fasciae

The pelvic fasciae consist of two main elements:

- The endopelvic fascia: It covers the pelvic floor muscles; it is continuous of the transversalis fascia and fuses with the hip bone's periosteum. The endopelvic fascia generally separates nerves going outside the pelvis (located on its outer side) from nerves innervating the inner pelvic organs (located on its inner side).
- The visceral fascia: It covers pelvic organs and constitutes also the perineural and perivascular sheaths.

Around the prostate, we can find three different fasciae. From outside to inside, we have the endopelvic fascia, the prostatic (visceral) fascia, and the Denonvilliers's fascia. The Denonvilliers's fascia is made up of connective tissue located between the posterior part of the prostate and the anterior part of the rectum. The fascia extends cranially toward the bladder neck, encompassing the seminal vesicles, and extends downward behind the prostate. The fascia thins as it descends to the external sphincter. Blood supply and autonomic innervation of the prostate are generally located between these three fascial layers (Fig. 1.2).

1.2.4 Sphincters

The urethral sphincter, which is composed of the internal and the external urethral sphincters, is crucial for maintaining urinary continence. It is also necessary for the ejaculatory process in males. Urethral sphincter injury is one of the most crucial contributing factors to post-radical prostatectomy urinary incontinence.

The internal sphincter is made of circular configuration of smooth muscle and is a continuum of the detrusor muscle of the bladder. It is located at the junction between the bladder neck and the urethra. It is supported, along with the bladder neck, by the pubovesical ligaments. It surrounds the preprostatic part of the urethra and encounters the prostate base in men. It is innervated by autonomous nervous fibers originating from the hypogastric plexus.

The external sphincter is located at the same level as the membranous urethra, distal to the internal sphincter, in the deep perineal pouch (between the pelvic diaphragm and the perineal membrane). It comprises circular skeletal muscle fibers that arise from the ischial rami, inferior pubic rami, and adjacent fascia. It is closely related to levator ani muscle and deep perineal and rectourethral muscles. The puboperineal fascicle of the levator ani muscle forms a circle around the external sphincter resulting therefore in a hiatus at the ventral aspect. It is innervated by the pudendal nerve.

These two sphincters are often considered as independent; however, anatomical research on cadavers has shown a certain degree of intricacy, and they are sometimes called altogether the "urethral sphincter complex."

1.2.5 Pelvic Floor Muscles

The pelvic diaphragm, which consists of the puborectalis, pubococcygeus, iliococcygeus, and coccygeus muscles, covers the entire lower pelvic outlet (Fig. 1.3). The puborectalis, pubococcygeus, and iliococcygeus form the levator ani muscle, and their function is to lift the pelvic floor upward and slightly forward. The pubococcygeus, iliococcygeus, and coccygeus muscles (all three have an insertion on the coccyx) constitute the flexors of the "tailbone" or coccyx. These muscles give access to two openings in men: the urethra anteriorly and the anus posteriorly. The pelvic diaphragm plays therefore an important role in assisting the sphincters in their continence action, as well as in the ejaculatory process. It also constitutes, along with pelvic fasciae described above, the primary support for the pelvic organs.

Below the pelvic diaphragm, another layer of muscles called the urogenital diaphragm, which consists of the superficial and deep transverse perineal muscles, covers the anterior half of the perineal diaphragm. These two muscles have a transverse orientation compared to muscles of the pelvic diaphragm which have generally an anteroposterior orientation. They support the pelvic floor and fix the perineal body, which consists of tendinous connective tissue and is considered as a crucial central anchor point for numerous pelvic floor muscles.

Finally, the bulbospongiosus and the ischiocavernosus muscles lie below the pelvic diaphragm and are the most superficial pelvic muscles. The bulbospongiosus surrounds the root of the penis and connects it to the perineal tendinous body. The ischiocavernosus interlaces with the penile root fascia and angles out to the ischial tuberosities. These two muscles attach and stabilize the penis. They also help in maintaining erection by compressing the penile veins and tensioning the connective tissue. The bulbospongiosus has also an additional role in expelling semen during ejaculation and emptying the urethra at the end of a micturition.

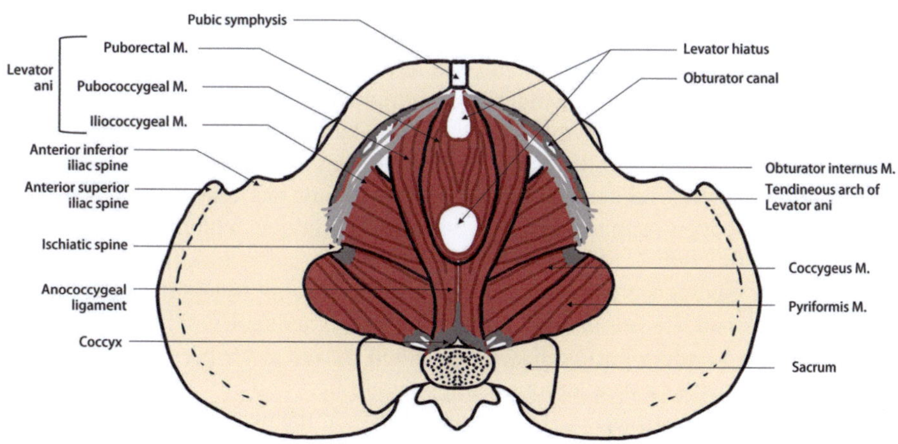

Fig. 1.3 Anatomy of the pelvic floor muscles. *M*. muscle

1.2.6 Nervous System

1.2.6.1 Pelvic Plexus

The pelvic plexus or inferior hypogastric plexus is the relay and integration center of the autonomous nerve fibers destined to the pelvic organs (bladder, prostate, uterus, and rectum) and erectile bodies. It is an even, lateral element located in the upper part of the ischiorectal fossa, within the thickness of the endopelvic fascia, on the lateral aspects of the rectum, posterior to the prostate, above and medial to the levator ani muscle. The pelvic plexus receives afferences from the sacral parasympathetic nucleus and the thoracolumbar and sacral sympathetic nucleus:

- The sympathetic system includes the hypogastric or prevertebral sympathetic pathway and the lumbosacral laterovertebral sympathetic pathway. The sympathetic branches arise from the gray matter of T11 to L2, cross the lumbar laterovertebral sympathetic ganglia, join branches arising from the preaortic plexuses (mesenteric, celiac), form the superior hypogastric plexus passing in front of the promontory, and then divide into an inverted Y joining the pelvic plexus. Other fibers pass through the laterovertebral lumbosacral sympathetic chain, located behind the large vessels, and join the cavernous nerves and the pelvic plexus.
- The parasympathetic center is located in the gray matter of S2, S3, and S4. The parasympathetic fibers travel through the anterior sacral roots and then through the cavernous nerves. They then anastomose with sympathetic nerve fibers from the sacral sympathetic ganglion chain to participate in the formation of the pelvic visceral nerves. These constitute the lower roots of the pelvic plexus. The sacral parasympathetic nerve fibers constitute the main erectile pathway.

1.2.6.2 Prostate Neuroanatomy

One of the most significant landmarks of prostate anatomy goes back to the works of Walsh et al. in 1982 [9]. The cavernous nerves are erectile nerves and arise from the lower part of the pelvic plexus between the rectum and the prostate just above the rectourethral muscle. Since they are not distinguishable macroscopically from their accompanying vascular elements, the term "neurovascular bundle" is usually used to refer to the structures isolated during radical prostatectomy with preservation of the erectile nerves. Within the neurovascular bundle, the nerves are usually located laterally to the vessels. Determining a flawless anatomical map of the neurovascular structures related to radical prostatectomy has emboldened surgeons with the knowledge to enhance the nerve-sparing technique, which is considered as important for functional recovery.

After their emergence from the lower part of the inferior hypogastric plexus, the neurovascular bundles are located posteriorly to the seminal vesicles, where they are susceptible to injury during dissection. When arrived at the periprostatic region, they become a network of interconnecting neural fibers and are arranged as a hammock in a trizonal distribution. The distance between the neurovascular bundle and the prostatic capsule is approximately 1.5 and 3 mm, respectively, at the prostatic base and at the apex. They are respectively located at 5 and 7 o'clock in relation to the prostatic urethra and at 3 and 9 o'clock in relation to the urethral sphincter. The distance between the nerves and the urethral lumen at this point is also small, and therefore, they are also susceptible to injury during dissection of the prostatic apex. In addition to the main neurovascular bundle, there are other smaller nerves, which are located and ramify in the prostatic fascia and Denonvilliers's fascia.

Recently, the concept of the neurovascular bundles has changed and they are now rather considered as a disperse assortment of structures that are not just restricted to the lateral edges of the Denonvilliers's fascia, but also extend medially to the midline, apart a gradually decreasing incidence of nerve fibers.

1.3 Modifications After Radical Prostatectomy

Removal of the prostate and seminal vesicles leads to major changes to the anatomy of the pelvic floor. The surgical excision of structures playing key functional roles and the anatomical reconfiguration induced by the vesicourethral anastomosis are the main causative agents in the pathophysiology of the most common postoperative complications of prostatectomy, namely, urinary incontinence, erectile dysfunction, penile shortening, bladder outlet obstruction, and inguinal hernias. Consequently, minimally invasive techniques for radical prostatectomy are constantly evolving aiming to achieve the best oncological outcomes while leaving most of the pelvic anatomy intact.

During prostatectomies, aside from inadvertent damage to the external urinary sphincter, the anterior and posterior structures constituting the main support to the urethra may be severed. The pubovesical and pubourethral ligaments and tendinous arch (white line) of the pelvic fascia play a major role in stabilizing the urethra and external urethral sphincter anteriorly to the pubic bone. Concurrently, the Denonvilliers's fascia, the anorectoperineal (rectourethral) muscle, and puborectalis fibers belonging to the levator ani muscle group are significant contributors to continence in view of their role in external compression of the membranous urethra during increases in abdominal pressure [10–12]. After surgery, concomitant damage of these structures alongside cephalad traction applied to the membranous urethra by the vesicourethral anastomosis determines significant changes in continence dynamics ultimately leading to a decreased urethral closure pressure and possibly stress urinary incontinence [13]. The decipherment of the complex multifactorial causes of post-prostatectomy urinary incontinence is being carried out simultaneously to several surgical modifications to limit a wide excision approach. Preservation of a longer membranous urethra as well as its preoperative length was associated to better continence outcomes in view of the intrinsic role of urethral fibers in determining the urethral closure pressure [14]. The Retzius-sparing approach was presented in 2010 as a feasible technique for transperitoneal robot-assisted prostatectomy through a single posterior incision at the level of the rectovesical pouch [5]. The complete preservation of the anterior support complex has been associated to higher urethral closure pressures especially by keeping anterior compression to the pubic bone in dynamic magnetic resonance imaging studies [15], with postoperative results showing enhanced early postoperative continence recovery and supporting the diffusion of this technique [16, 17]. In non-Retzius-sparing approaches, preservation and reconstruction techniques have been proposed to reestablish pelvic dynamics similar to the preoperative state, with some randomized-controlled trials supporting the effectiveness of such techniques. Preservation of the puboprostatic collar and anterior suspension on the bladder neck to the tendinous arch were shown to be significant contributors to postoperative continence, with highly promising results shown by several surgical modifications to robot-assisted prostatectomy including the novel "hood technique" introduced in 2020 and intended to achieve total anatomical preservation of the anterior support complex despite using a traditional anterior approach [7]. Posterior reconstruction of the striated sphincter was first described in 2007 as a simple surgical implementation to reestablish the continuity of the sphincter and the Denonvilliers's fascia and overall reinstate the dynamic external compression function carried out by the posterior musculofascial plate [18]. Randomized-controlled trials (RCT) have shown improved continence outcomes of posterior reconstructions as well as of a combination of anterior and posterior techniques, although these results were not confirmed in all RCTs and the evidence of the added benefit of reconstruction techniques to continence remains equivocal [19–23]. Ultimately, urinary incontinence has also been linked to the extent of periprostatic nerve damage during surgery. As a matter of fact, improved early continence outcomes were observed in patients receiving higher grades of nerve sparing due to a possible preservation of the nerve supply of the membranous urethra and external sphincter [24]. Denervation has a less clear role in the onset of postoperative bladder dysfunction as a concurrent cause of urinary incontinence, and it has been advocated as a possible cause for de novo overactive bladder syndrome with or without urinary incontinence in open retropubic prostatectomy [25]. A urethrogenic mechanism related to a decreased urethral tone after prostatectomy may also be an underlying cause of postoperative detrusor overactivity as leakage of urine in the urethra due to stress incontinence may trigger the micturition reflex through urethral afferent nerves [26]. The urethrogenic theory and the role of denervation are also supported by a prospective assessment of the onset of detrusor overactivity in patients undergoing robot-assisted prostatectomy, with a statistically significant higher maximum urethral closure pressures and degree of nerve sparing reported in patients free of overactive bladder syndrome after surgery [27].

Some degree of periprostatic nerve damage due to transection, traction, or cautery during prostatectomy is unavoidable, as modern morphological analysis confirmed a widespread "mesh-like" distribution of the periprostatic nerve plexus from the anterior to the posterolateral area of the gland [4, 28]. Beginning with the pioneering work of Walsh et al. in 1980s, surgical damage of the periprostatic fibers responsible for the integrated neurovascular response controlling potency has traditionally been identified as the main cause for post-prostatectomy erectile dysfunction (ED) [9]. A progressive narrowing of the surgical excision margins of prostatectomy to include "nerve-sparing" (NS) techniques has subsequently confirmed the etiology of post-prostatectomy ED, and minimally invasive approaches such as laparoscopy or robot assistance have catalyzed the implementation of bilateral NS in the standard surgical practice for localized prostate cancer [29, 30]. Research in nerve distribution and periprostatic anatomy has led to the acknowledgment of fascial planes and different degrees of posterolateral NS (Table 1.1) [31, 32], with intrafascial approaches showing the best erectile and continence recovery rates while preserving adequate control of surgical margins [33]. Although only a minor quota of parasympathetic fibers runs within the anterolateral portion of the periprostatic plexus, different NS techniques offering a low-traction anterolateral preservation of the plexus have shown promising rates of potency recovery, including the 2020 retrograde release approach [34] and the 2009 Vattikuti Institute-modified superveil technique, an anterolateral dissection technique intended to preserve the lateral periprostatic fascia, the pubovesical ligaments, and the dorsal vein complex to offer complete anterolateral NS [35]. Thermal injury due to activation of energy sources in proximity to the periprostatic plexus has traditionally been identified as one of the leading causes of nerve damage [36]. Despite this, precise low-energy bipolar coagulation adjacent to the plexus was shown to offer potency and continence recovery similar to energy-free NS. Prospective trials investigating this aspect are still lacking [37]. NS techniques remain a developing field of surgical research, and while a considerable effort is spent in the refinement of the understanding of post-prostatectomy ED, the intent to narrow the surgical excision plains to allow maximal NS while retaining excellent cancer control has led to the

Table 1.1 Key histological and anatomical landmarks for nerve-sparing radical prostatectomy

Landmark	Role in nerve-sparing (NS) radical prostatectomy
Prostatic fascia	Thin connective layer covering the posterolateral aspect of the prostatic capsule
Denonvilliers's fascia (DF)	Multilayered connective tissue located between the posterior aspect of the prostate and the rectum
Landmark artery (LA)	Pericapsular arterial vessel running along the posterolateral aspect of the prostate, medially to most of the nerve trunks. A progressive NS grading system (Grades 5 to 1) centered on the LA has been proposed [32]
Pearly areolar tissue	Thin fatty plane between the LA and the prostatic fascia. Grade 5 (>95%) NS is performed on the plane between the prostatic fascia and pearly areolar tissue, while Grade 4 (75%) near complete NS is performed on a plane between the LA and pearly areolar tissue. Grades 3–2 planes are identified by NS increasingly lateral to the LA
Venous plane (VP)	Pericapsular venous plexus running along the posterolateral aspect of the prostate. A progressive nerve-sparing grading system (Grades I to IV) centered on the VP has been proposed [31]. Grade I (complete) NS is performed on the medial VP with minimal incision of the DF. Grade II NS is performed on a perivenous plane by incising the uppermost layer of the DF. Grade III (partial/incremental) NS is performed through an incision of the neural and adipose tissue laterally to the VP sacrificing the medial nerve trunks
Levator ani muscle fascia	Connective layer covering the levator ani muscle complex laterally to the neurovascular bundle. The appropriate plane of dissection for wide-excision Grade 1/IV non-NS radical prostatectomy is identified between the levator ani muscle fascia and the neurovascular bundle

proposal of the “precision prostatectomy” protocol, a novel surgical technique involving removal of all of the gland except for a 5–10 mm rim of the capsule contralateral to the dominant cancer lesion. A randomized control trial on this technique is currently being conducted, and its results might further expand the understanding of anatomical modifications leading to post-prostatectomy ED [38, 39].

Penile length shortening (PLS) is an immediate and often temporary finding consequential to prostate removal and formation of the vesicourethral anastomosis. A cross-sectional study of 1422 patients receiving radical prostatectomy has shown a 55% rate of self-perceived postoperative PLS compared to when the patients were 30 years old. PLS rates were significantly lower at 26% in an age-matched cohort identified in the general population [40]. Overall PLS is a very common occurrence experiences by up to 70% patients receiving a radical prostatectomy, with shortening often greater than 1 cm in stretched penile length [41]. Postoperative erectile function and anatomical changes were identified as the main factors contributing to the etiology of PLS. A prospective analysis of recovery patterns in 352 patients at 1 year after prostatectomy has shown complete recovery of stretched penile length in 60.2% of cases and a mean PLS of 16.4% (2.36 cm) in patients experiencing incomplete recovery. Consistent use of phosphodiesterase type 5 inhibitors was significantly associated to complete length recovery [42]. The evidence on the role of nerve sparing in reducing PLS is to date inconclusive [43]. Cephalad-oriented tension exerted by the vesical pedicles determining a vertical retraction of the integrated structure constituted by the membranous urethra, urogenital diaphragm, and bulb of the penis was identified as the main anatomical cause of PLS in a magnetic resonance imaging analysis. The study assessed 102 patients receiving radical prostatectomy and correlated these anatomical changes to a maximal PLS at 10 days postoperatively. Gradual recovery to preoperative length at 12 months was observed and matched by the return of the bulb of the penis to almost the same preoperative position, possibly due to a progressive loosening of the tension of the vascular pedicles [43].

Vesicourethral anastomosis stenosis (VAUS) is a common cause of bladder outlet obstruction usually ensuing within the first 24 months after radical prostatectomy [44]. Incidence rates were shown to correlate to surgical invasiveness in modern series of 17,299 patients receiving a prostatectomy in the United Kingdom, with surgical reintervention rates for VAUS within 2 years of prostatectomy of 3.3% for robot-assisted approaches, 5.7% for laparoscopic approaches, and 6.9% for open retropubic cases [45]. Several patient-specific factors correlating to decreased local microvasculature, dysfunctional healing, and luminal constriction have been associated to the etiology of VAUS, including higher disease burden and prostate volume, cardiovascular comorbidities, diabetes mellitus, obesity, smoking, previous bladder outlet obstruction surgery, and older age. Surgery-related factors were also identified as covariates to VAUS onset, with wide excision prostatectomy, perianastomotic urinoma/hematoma, and length of surgery being significantly associated to the risk of VAUS [46, 47]. Catheter diameter was also shown to correlate with VAUS rates in an analysis of 1000 consecutive RALPs, with significantly lower stenosis rates observed for 16–18 Ch vs 22 Ch catheters, possibly due to lower intraluminal pressures on the mucosal wall during the healing process [48]. Single-knot running sutures have gained popularity in minimally invasive prostatectomy as a simple anastomotic technique achieving adequate mucosal apposition in water-tight non-ischemic anastomosis [49, 50]. Accrued evidence has shown the advantages of running over interrupted sutures in view of shorter anastomosis times and lower extravasation rates, although long-term differences for VAUS rates were nonsignificant among the two approaches [51].

Indirect inguinal hernia (IH) is a frequent complication occurring within 2–3 years from radical prostatectomy [52], most probably caused by a postoperative contraction of the abdominal layers at the level of the medial inguinal fossa (Hesselbach's triangle), which receive surgical insult during the development of the Retzius' space. Such contraction could in turn cause a retraction and consecutive weaking of the internal inguinal ring, leading to a diathesis to herniation [53]. This etiological hypothesis is supported by a retrospective analysis of 839 patients receiving a prostatectomy either through a conventional anterior or Retzius-sparing approach, with data showing that patients receiving a surgical insult at the level of the Retzius' space had an hazard ratio of 2.8 (95% CI 1.5–5.5) for inguinal hernia formation [54]. Patients with a BMI <25 were also found to be at higher risk for inguinal hernia formation compared to a reference set at BMI ≥25 [54]. Surgical invasiveness was also shown to directly correlate to inguinal hernia incidence in a meta-analysis of 54 studies for a total of 101,687 patients, with an IH incidence of 13.7% (95% CI 12.0–15.4) in open retropubic cases, 7.5% (95% CI 5.2–9.8) in laparoscopic cases, and 7.9% (95% CI 5.0–10.9) with a robot-assisted approach [52]. Several studies proposed prophylactic techniques to prevent IH including the isolation of the spermatic cord from the internal inguinal ring with or without subsequent dissection of the vas deferens from the spermatic cord. When identified, dissection and ligation of the processus vaginalis was also included in this approach. Overall, IH prevention techniques were shown to decrease the risk of postoperative IH [52].

1.4 Modifications After Male Cystectomy

Radical cystectomy is a major surgical procedure that involves removal of the urinary bladder, the prostate, and the pelvic lymph nodes in men. The procedure results in major modifications of the pelvic anatomy and physiopathology with consequences on sexual function and urinary continence, in case of neobladder reconstruction.

Regarding neurovascular anatomy, the main damage during surgery can occur during prostatic dissection, as discussed in the previous paragraph. The main difference during radical cystectomy is that the vascular control and dissection begins at the level of the superior vesical artery and follows caudally toward the prostatic plexus. In this anatomical segment (between the superior vesical artery and the prostatic artery), the neurovascular bundle lies close and can be damaged in case of excessive traction, exaggerated use of diathermy, and extensive dissection, as in the case of locally advanced disease. In patients who are candidates for a nerve-sparing radical cystectomy according to preoperative sexual function and stage of bladder cancer, care must be taken during vascular control of the vesical pedicle. We advise cautious use of cautery, in favor of surgical clips to avoid thermal damage to the neurovascular bundle. In order to define the adequate level of control and avoid too extensive dissection, we advise to identify early the tip of the seminal vesicles and prostatic base and trying to follow the bladder vasculature to that point. The blood supply to the seminal vesicles should also be controlled with clips, adjacent to the organ to avoid neurovascular damage.

Pelvic lymph node dissection (PLND) is a mandatory and integrative step of radical cystectomy [55]. The extent of the dissection is still a matter of debate across the surgical community, although the only available randomized controlled trial found no true benefit of extending the dissection above the iliac bifurcation [56]. In patients for whom the dissection is carried out up to the aortic bifurcation, including the presacral nodes, surgeons must be aware of the potential damage to parasympathetic nerve fibers during such surgical step [57]. As such, given the absence of a proven oncologic advantage, for patients undergoing nerve-sparing radical cystectomy, we advocate against presacral node dissection, maintaining the ureteral crossing as upper limit.

Regarding preservation of continence in case of neobladder reconstruction, the key concepts of prostatic surgery apply to radical cystectomy. Maximal urethral length preservation is paramount. Given the possibility of resecting the prostate in an intrafascial plane without major oncologic risks, surgeons must really maximize apical dissection and consequent urethral length. Reconstruction of the posterior plane as in radical prostatectomy should be implemented in order to increase posterior urethral support and reduce traction on the urethra [58].

1.5 Conclusions

Pelvic anatomy is complex, and its knowledge is constantly evolving, thanks to new surgical techniques, and enhanced by improved surgical imaging. Apart from pure prostatic and vesical anatomy, surgeons must understand the support structures surrounding these organs as well as the deep neurovascular anatomy. The anterior support to the urinary sphincter and bladder has seen an upsurge in its importance after the development of the Retzius-sparing approach and the publication of its excellent urinary continence rates. Sexual preservation after radical cystectomy is today recommended is sexually active men and requires knowledge of the anatomy of the neurovascular bundle and autonomic nervous plexus during extended PLND.

References

1. Catto JWF, Mandrik O, Quayle LA, et al. Diagnosis, treatment and survival from bladder, upper urinary tract and urethral cancers: real world findings from NHS England between 2013 and 2019. BJU Int. 2023;131:734. https://doi.org/10.1111/bju.15970.
2. Albisinni S, Joniau S, Quackels T, et al. Current trends in patient enrollment for robotic-assisted laparoscopic prostatectomy in Belgium. Cancer. 2017;123:4139–46.

3. Schuessler WW, Schulam PG, Clayman RV, Kavoussi LR. Laparoscopic radical prostatectomy: initial short-term experience. Urology. 1997;50:854–7.
4. Walz J, Epstein JI, Ganzer R, et al. A critical analysis of the current knowledge of surgical anatomy of the prostate related to optimisation of cancer control and preservation of continence and erection in candidates for radical prostatectomy: an update. Eur Urol. 2016;70:301–11.
5. Galfano A, Ascione A, Grimaldi S, Petralia G, Strada E, Bocciardi AM. A new anatomic approach for robot-assisted laparoscopic prostatectomy: a feasibility study for completely intrafascial surgery. Eur Urol. 2010;58:457–61.
6. Asimakopoulos AD, Mugnier C, Hoepffner J-L, Piechaud T, Gaston R. Bladder neck preservation during minimally invasive radical prostatectomy: a standardised technique using a lateral approach. BJU Int. 2012;110:1566–71.
7. Wagaskar VG, Mittal A, Sobotka S, et al. Hood technique for robotic radical prostatectomy—preserving periurethral anatomical structures in the space of Retzius and sparing the pouch of Douglas, enabling early return of continence without compromising surgical margin rates. Eur Urol. 2021;80:213–21.
8. Seetharam Bhat KR, Moschovas MC, Sandri M, et al. Stratification of potency outcomes following robot-assisted laparoscopic radical prostatectomy based on age, preoperative potency, and nerve sparing. J Endourol. 2021;35:1631–8.
9. Walsh PC, Donker PJ. Impotence following radical prostatectomy: insight into etiology and prevention. J Urol. 1982;128:492–7.
10. Steiner MS. The puboprostatic ligament and the male urethral suspensory mechanism: an anatomic study. Urology. 1994;44:530–4.
11. Burnett AL, Mostwin JL. In situ anatomical study of the male urethral sphincteric complex: relevance to continence preservation following major pelvic surgery. J Urol. 1998;160:1301–6.
12. Steiner MS. Anatomic basis for the continence-preserving radical retropubic prostatectomy. Semin Urol Oncol. 2000;18:9–18.
13. Kadono Y, Nohara T, Kawaguchi S, et al. Investigating the mechanism underlying urinary continence recovery after radical prostatectomy: effectiveness of a longer urethral stump to prevent urinary incontinence. BJU Int. 2018;122:456–62.
14. Mungovan SF, Sandhu JS, Akin O, Smart NA, Graham PL, Patel MI. Preoperative membranous urethral length measurement and continence recovery following radical prostatectomy: a systematic review and meta-analysis. Eur Urol. 2017;71:368–78.
15. Kadono Y, Nohara T, Kawaguchi S, et al. Investigating the mechanism underlying urinary continence using dynamic MRI after Retzius-sparing robot-assisted radical prostatectomy. Sci Rep. 2022;12:3975.
16. Albisinni S, Dasnoy C, Diamand R, Mjaess G, Aoun F, Esperto F, Porpiglia F, Fiori C, Roumeguere T, De Nunzio C. Anterior vs. Retzius-sparing robotic assisted radical prostatectomy: can the approach really make a difference? Minerva Urol Nephrol. 2022;74:137. https://doi.org/10.23736/S2724-6051.21.04623-1.
17. Checcucci E, Veccia A, Fiori C, et al. Retzius-sparing robot-assisted radical prostatectomy vs the standard approach: a systematic review and analysis of comparative outcomes. BJU Int. 2020;125:8–16.
18. Rocco F, Carmignani L, Acquati P, Gadda F, Dell'Orto P, Rocco B, Casellato S, Gazzano G, Consonni D. Early continence recovery after open radical prostatectomy with restoration of the posterior aspect of the rhabdosphincter. Eur Urol. 2007;52:376–83.
19. Hurtes X, Rouprêt M, Vaessen C, Pereira H, Faivre d'Arcier B, Cormier L, Bruyère F. Anterior suspension combined with posterior reconstruction during robot-assisted laparoscopic prostatectomy improves early return of urinary continence: a prospective randomized multicentre trial: anterior suspension combined with posterior reconstruction. BJU Int. 2012;110:875–83.
20. Koliakos N, Mottrie A, Buffi N, De Naeyer G, Willemsen P, Fonteyne E. Posterior and anterior fixation of the urethra during robotic prostatectomy improves early continence rates. Scand J Urol Nephrol. 2010;44:5–10.
21. Salazar A, Regis L, Planas J, Celma A, Santamaria A, Trilla E, Morote J. A randomised controlled trial to assess the benefit of posterior rhabdosphincter reconstruction in early urinary continence recovery after robot-assisted radical prostatectomy. Eur Urol Oncol. 2022;5:460–3.

22. Jeong CW, Lee JK, Oh JJ, Lee S, Jeong SJ, Hong SK, Byun S-S, Lee SE. Effects of new 1-step posterior reconstruction method on recovery of continence after robot-assisted laparoscopic prostatectomy: results of a prospective, single-blind, parallel group, randomized, controlled trial. J Urol. 2015;193:935–42.
23. Sutherland DE, Linder B, Guzman AM, Hong M, Frazier HA, Engel JD, Bianco FJ. Posterior rhabdosphincter reconstruction during robotic assisted radical prostatectomy: results from a phase II randomized clinical trial. J Urol. 2011;185:1262–7.
24. Reeves F, Preece P, Kapoor J, Everaerts W, Murphy DG, Corcoran NM, Costello AJ. Preservation of the neurovascular bundles is associated with improved time to continence after radical prostatectomy but not long-term continence rates: results of a systematic review and meta-analysis. Eur Urol. 2015;68:692–704.
25. Porena M, Mearini E, Mearini L, Vianello A, Giannantoni A. Voiding dysfunction after radical retropubic prostatectomy: more than external urethral sphincter deficiency. Eur Urol. 2007;52:38–45.
26. Jung SY, Fraser MO, Ozawa H, Yokoyama O, Yoshiyama M, De Groat WC, Chancellor MB. Urethral afferent nerve activity affects the micturition reflex; implication for the relationship between stress incontinence and detrusor instability. J Urol. 1999;162:204–12.
27. Matsukawa Y, Yoshino Y, Ishida S, Fujita T, Majima T, Funahashi Y, Sassa N, Kato M, Gotoh M. De novo overactive bladder after robot-assisted laparoscopic radical prostatectomy. Neurourol Urodyn. 2018;37:2008–14.
28. Sievert K-D, Hennenlotter J, Dillenburg T, Toomey P, Wöllner J, Zweers P, Pannek J, Andersson K-E, Amend B. Extended periprostatic nerve distributions on the prostate surface confirmed using diffusion tensor imaging. BJU Int. 2019;123:995–1004.
29. Kyriazis I, Spinos T, Tsaturyan A, Kallidonis P, Stolzenburg JU, Liatsikos E. Different nerve-sparing techniques during radical prostatectomy and their impact on functional outcomes. Cancers. 2022;14:1601.
30. Avulova S, Zhao Z, Lee D, et al. The effect of nerve sparing status on sexual and urinary function: 3-year results from the CEASAR study. J Urol. 2018;199:1202–9.
31. Tewari AK, Srivastava A, Huang MW, et al. Anatomical grades of nerve sparing: a risk-stratified approach to neural-hammock sparing during robot-assisted radical prostatectomy (RARP). BJU Int. 2011;108:984–92.
32. Schatloff O, Chauhan S, Sivaraman A, Kameh D, Palmer KJ, Patel VR. Anatomic grading of nerve sparing during robot-assisted radical prostatectomy. Eur Urol. 2012;61:796–802.
33. Weng H, Zeng X-T, Li S, Meng X-Y, Shi M-J, He D-L, Wang X-H. Intrafascial versus interfascial nerve sparing in radical prostatectomy for localized prostate cancer: a systematic review and meta-analysis. Sci Rep. 2017;7:11454.
34. de Carvalho PA, Barbosa JABA, Guglielmetti GB, Cordeiro MD, Rocco B, Nahas WC, Patel V, Coelho RF. Retrograde release of the neurovascular bundle with preservation of dorsal venous complex during robot-assisted radical prostatectomy: optimizing functional outcomes. Eur Urol. 2020;77:628–35.
35. Menon M, Shrivastava A, Bhandari M, Satyanarayana R, Siva S, Agarwal PK. Vattikuti Institute prostatectomy: technical modifications in 2009. Eur Urol. 2009;56:89–96.
36. Ong AM, Su L-M, Varkarakis I, Inagaki T, Link RE, Bhayani SB, Patriciu A, Crain B, Walsh PC. Nerve sparing radical prostatectomy: effects of hemostatic energy sources on the recovery of cavernous nerve function in a canine model. J Urol. 2004;172:1318–22.
37. de la Taille A. Nerve-sparing techniques during robot-assisted radical prostatectomy: clips or low-energy bipolar coagulation? Low energy. Eur Urol Open Sci. 2022;44:102–3.
38. Sood A, Abdollah F, Jeong W, Menon M. The precision prostatectomy: "waiting for Godot". Eur Urol Focus. 2020;6:227–30.
39. Pedraza AM, Wagaskar V, Parekh S, Tewari A. Technical advances in nerve-sparing and continence preservation. Curr Opin Urol. 2022;32:204–10.
40. Carlsson S, Nilsson AE, Johansson E, Nyberg T, Akre O, Steineck G. Self-perceived penile shortening after radical prostatectomy. Int J Impot Res. 2012;24:179–84.

41. Frey AU, Sønksen J, Fode M. Neglected side effects after radical prostatectomy: a systematic review. J Sex Med. 2014;11:374–85.
42. Kwon YS, Farber N, Yu JW, et al. Longitudinal recovery patterns of penile length and the underexplored benefit of long-term phosphodiesterase-5 inhibitor use after radical prostatectomy. BMC Urol. 2018;18:37.
43. Kadono Y, Machioka K, Nakashima K, et al. Changes in penile length after radical prostatectomy: investigation of the underlying anatomical mechanism. BJU Int. 2017;120:293–9.
44. Herschorn S, Elliott S, Coburn M, Wessells H, Zinman L. SIU/ICUD consultation on urethral strictures: posterior urethral stenosis after treatment of prostate cancer. Urology. 2014;83:S59–70.
45. Sujenthiran A, Nossiter J, Parry M, Charman SC, Aggarwal A, Payne H, Dasgupta P, Clarke NW, van der Meulen J, Cathcart P. National cohort study comparing severe medium-term urinary complications after robot-assisted vs laparoscopic vs retropubic open radical prostatectomy. BJU Int. 2018;121:445–52.
46. Rocco NR, Zuckerman JM. An update on best practice in the diagnosis and management of post-prostatectomy anastomotic strictures. Ther Adv Urol. 2017;9:99–110.
47. Nicholson HL, Al-Hakeem Y, Maldonado JJ, Tse V. Management of bladder neck stenosis and urethral stricture and stenosis following treatment for prostate cancer. Transl Androl Urol. 2017;6:S92–S102.
48. Liss MA, Skarecky D, Morales B, Osann K, Eichel L, Ahlering TE. Preventing perioperative complications of robotic-assisted radical prostatectomy. Urology. 2013;81:319–23.
49. Albisinni S, Aoun F, Peltier A, van Velthoven R. The single-knot running vesicourethral anastomosis after minimally invasive prostatectomy: review of the technique and its modifications, tips, and pitfalls. Prostate Cancer. 2016;2016:1–5.
50. Albisinni S, Limani K, Hawaux E, Peltier A, Van Velthoven R. Evaluation of the single-knot running vesicourethral anastomosis 10 years after its introduction: results from an international survey. J Laparoendosc Adv Surg Tech. 2014;24:640–6.
51. Kowalewski KF, Tapking C, Hetjens S, Nickel F, Mandel P, Nuhn P, Ritter M, Moul JW, Thüroff JW, Kriegmair MC. Interrupted versus continuous suturing for vesicourethral anastomosis during radical prostatectomy: a systematic review and meta-analysis. Eur Urol Focus. 2019;5:980–91.
52. Alder R, Zetner D, Rosenberg J. Incidence of inguinal hernia after radical prostatectomy: a systematic review and meta-analysis. J Urol. 2020;203:265–74.
53. Kadono Y, Nohara T, Kawaguchi S, et al. Novel prevention procedure for inguinal hernia after robot-assisted radical prostatectomy: results from a prospective randomized trial. J Endourol. 2019;33:302–8.
54. Chang KD, Abdel Raheem A, Santok GDR, Kim LHC, Lum TGH, Lee SH, Ham WS, Choi YD, Rha KH. Anatomical Retzius-space preservation is associated with lower incidence of postoperative inguinal hernia development after robot-assisted radical prostatectomy. Hernia. 2017;21:555–61.
55. Witjes JA, Bruins HM, Cathomas R, et al. European Association of Urology guidelines on muscle-invasive and metastatic bladder cancer: summary of the 2020 guidelines. Eur Urol. 2021;79:82–104.
56. Gschwend JE, Heck MM, Lehmann J, et al. Extended versus limited lymph node dissection in bladder cancer patients undergoing radical cystectomy: survival results from a prospective, randomized trial. Eur Urol. 2019;75:604–11.
57. Shiozawa T, Huebner M, Hirt B, Wallwiener D, Reisenauer C. Nerve-preserving sacrocolpopexy: anatomical study and surgical approach. Eur J Obstet Gynecol Reprod Biol. 2010;152:103–7.
58. Rocco B, Assumma S, Calcagnile T, Sangalli M, Turri F, Micali S, Gaia G, Bozzini G, Sighinolfi MC. Reproducibility of a modified posterior reconstruction during robotic intracorporeal neobladder reconfiguration. Int Braz J Urol. 2022;49:136–42.

Preventing Urinary and Sexual Dysfunctions After Prostatectomy: Surgical Tips and Tricks

2

Paolo Minafra, Luciano Rella, Salvatore Gerbasi, and Marco Spilotros

2.1 Introduction

Radical prostatectomy is the standard surgical treatment for localized prostate cancer [1]. The ideal treatment of localized prostate cancer would provide complete tumor eradication while warranting a low risk of complications and excellent functional results, particularly referring to continence and erectile function preservation.

The etiology of erectile dysfunction and urinary incontinence after radical prostatectomy is complex and multifactorial. These factors encompass anatomical and surgical aspects, but also patient characteristics, such as age, body mass index, large prostatic volume, lower urinary tract symptoms, and preoperative continence level [2, 3].

Furthermore, since the introduction of Walsh's radical prostatectomy in 1987, which described the fundamental landmarks for the "modern" radical prostatectomy [4], several efforts have been made to improve the surgical technique in order to achieve all these goals.

Nowadays, state of the art is represented by robot-assisted laparoscopic prostatectomy (RALP) [5]. Advantages of the robotic system include improved ergonomics, and wristed instrumentation facilitates suturing and dissection during minimally invasive prostatectomy [6]. Therefore, robotic assistance made easier the application of Walsh's principles to laparoscopic prostatectomy and allowed the deepening

P. Minafra
Mater Dei Hospital, Bari, Italy

L. Rella · S. Gerbasi · M. Spilotros (✉)
Department of Emergency and Organ Transplantation—Urology, Andrology and Kidney Transplantation Unit, University of Bari, Bari, Italy
e-mail: marco.spilotros@uniba.it

G. Lamberti, C. De Nunzio (eds.), *Bladder, Bowel and Sexual Dysfunctions Rehabilitation after Radical Prostatectomy*, Urodynamics, Neurourology and Pelvic Floor Dysfunctions, https://doi.org/10.1007/978-3-031-76341-0_2

of urologists' awareness of anatomical details and the development of new surgical strategies [7].

Moreover, the widespread diffusion of the robotic surgery, with its magnified, three-dimensional visualization, gave a great contribution to the development of a deeper anatomical insight on prostate and its surrounding pelvic structures [8]. The better confidence with periprostatic anatomy allows a more anatomical approach to radical prostatectomy and the tailoring of the procedure according to cancer characteristics, in order to improve functional result while warranting the oncological safety [9].

2.2 Surgical and Functional Anatomy

2.2.1 Prevesical Space and Puboprostatic Complex

The prevesical space of Retzius is the extraperitoneal region between the pubis and the bladder and the prostate. It is filled with fibrofatty tissue and contains the structures of the puboprostatic complex that are responsible for the anterior attachment of prostate and proximal urethra to the pubic symphysis [10, 11] (Fig. 2.1).

The main elements of the puboprostatic complex are (a) puboprostatic ligaments, which arise from the posteroinferior surface of the pubis and reach the anterolateral prostatic face, in proximity to the apex; (b) dorsal venous complex (DVC); (c) anterior detrusor apron, fibromuscular connective tissue originating from the longitudinal smooth muscle of the bladder and extending anteriorly toward the pubis; and (d) pubourethral ligament.

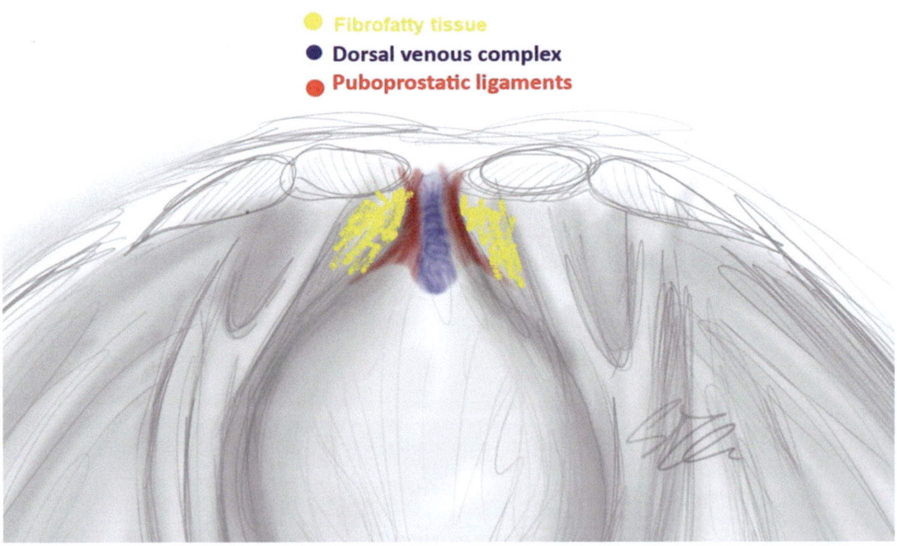

Fig. 2.1 Graphical representation of the prevesical space of Retzius

2.2.2 Prostatic Fasciae

The nomenclature of periprostatic fascial structures lacks standardization [12]. Even though, a few main fascial structures are generally identified around the prostate.

The endopelvic fascia is a sheet of connective tissue that continues from the transversalis fascia and runs on pelvic walls and floor covering the obturator internus, piriformis, levator ani, and coccygeus muscles. On the lateral wall of the pelvis, it thickens in the tendinous arch of pelvic fascia and splits in two layers: The parietal layer, also named lateral pelvic fascia, covers the pelvic floor muscles (also referred to as levator ani fascia). The other runs medially to envelop the pelvic organs and takes the name of visceral pelvic fascia [13].

The periprostatic fascia (or prostatic fascia) is the visceral pelvic fascia extending immediately around the prostate. Usually, it is not a discrete structure but a multilayered organization of collagenous and adipose tissue elements over the prostate. It is closely attached to the fibromuscular stroma of the so-called prostatic capsule, especially on the anterior and posterior midline (the prostate has not an actual capsule but a fibromuscular tissue that constitutes the outer layer of the gland and is an extension of the underlying prostatic stroma). On the posterior surface of the prostate, it is medially fused with the Denonvilliers' fascia, but moving mediolaterally, these two layers separate [5].

The posterior periprostatic fascia (also universally called as Denonvilliers' fascia) is located in the rectoprostatic space. Its upper part is a continuous layer and covers the seminal vesicles and the posterior prostatic surface. As it extends caudally, it becomes thinner and reaches the apex of the prostate [12] (Fig. 2.2).

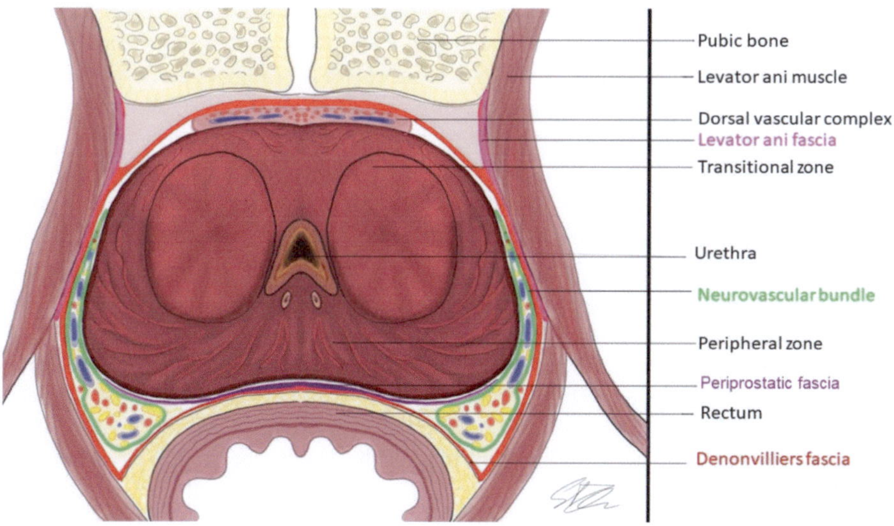

Fig. 2.2 Graphical representation of the prostate and its relation with fascial structures of the pelvis

The embryological origin of Denonvilliers' fascia is debated. Some authors believe it is formed by obliteration of the vesicorectal pouch of the peritoneum [14]. For this reason, this band would have an anterior and a posterior layer. More recently, it has been clarified that the Denonvilliers' fascia layers are not separable and that what many wrongly called as "posterior layer of the Denonvilliers' fascia" is actually the ventral rectal fascia. This fascia descends in front of the rectum and melts with the perineal body [15, 16].

Posterolaterally to the prostate, the lateral prostatic fascia, the Denonvilliers' fascia, and the levator ani fascia delimit a triangular space. The blood supply and the autonomic innervation to the prostate mainly run between these layers.

2.2.3 Periprostatic Neuroanatomy

In the male, the inferior hypogastric plexus or pelvic plexus is responsible for the mechanisms of erection, ejaculation, and urinary continence [17, 18]. Anatomical studies on cadaveric models have shown that pelvic splanchnic nerves contain parasympathetic fibers (including those for erigentes nerves) that originate from the ventral rami of S2–S4 but also contains up to 36% sympathetic fibers that derive from the hypogastric nerve originating mainly from T11 to L2 and responsible for ejaculation [19]. Consequently, the nerves in the aforementioned areas could also contribute to urinary continence in addition to erectile function [20].

Urologists' conception of the anatomy of periprostatic nervous structures has evolved from the Walsh and Donker's classical concept of a "cord-like" neurovascular bundles [21] containing the cavernous nerve [18].

More recently, the "trizonal" concept has been developed from contemporary anatomical studies. According to this new vision, there are three zones of neural tissue to mind during radical prostatectomy. Even if there is no uniformity in the nomenclature of these neural zones, this concept is nowadays shared by different authors. Herein, we report the nomenclature proposed by Tewari [22]: (a) Proximal neurovascular plate (PNP) is a wide area of neural fibers arising from the pelvic splanchnic nerve over the lateral rectal fascia and extended laterally to the bladder neck and the seminal vesicles. Some of these fibers converge into the cavernous nerve. (b) Predominant neurovascular bundle (PNB) represents the distal continuation of the PNP. It matches with the classical definition of NVB and runs on the posterolateral aspect of the prostate. (c) The accessory distal neural pathways (ANP) are supplementary neural ways formed by fibers that remain divergent over the lateral prostatic fascia, even if their role in erectile function remains debatable [23]. According to some authors, they are localized on the anterolateral and the posterior aspect of the prostate [24]. Others described an apical plexus on the posterolateral aspect of the prostatic apex and urethra that might be present in 35% of men [18].

The nerve fibers that form the cavernous nerves more distally course onto the lateral surface of the membranous urethra before penetrating the urogenital diaphragm to reach the corpora cavernosa.

2.3 Neurovascular Bundles Preservation

Preservation of the neurovascular bundles (NVB) plays a crucial role in potency recovery after radical prostatectomy and has also been demonstrated to be associated with better continence rates [25, 26]. In order to perform a high degree of NVB preservation, the dissection planes are closer to the prostate than in non-sparing technique, consequently increasing the risk of positive surgical margins (PSM) [27].

The medial or lateral plane of dissection of the prostatic arteries represents the main landmark to preserve the NVB. The grades of dissection may vary from grade 1 (no nerve sparing) to 5 (≥95% of nerve sparing) [28]. Nerve-sparing techniques can be distinguished based on the fascial planes of dissection (intrafascial, interfascial, or extrafascial) and the direction of dissection (retrograde or antegrade). In the last decades, especially with the advent of robotic surgery [29], several techniques and approaches have been proposed in order to minimize NVB injuries, thus optimizing maintenance of erectile function and achievement of a radical resection.

2.3.1 Planes of Dissection

2.3.1.1 The Extrafascial Dissection

This dissection is performed under Denonvilliers' fascia, as evidenced by the presence of perirectal fat on the posterior aspect of the dissection plane. The extrafascial plane of dissection is located laterally to the prostatic fascia and is associated with complete NVB removal and the worst postoperative potency and continence recovery. However, in terms of oncologic dissection, it is the safest and most indicated in patients with pT3 disease [30].

2.3.1.2 The Interfascial Dissection

In the interfascial nerve-sparing approach, the prostatic fascia is retained intact and dissection is performed within the plane between the prostatic fascia and the lateral pelvic fascia. When entering this space, the lateral prostatic fascia is resected and remains attached to the final specimen. Although the original procedure described by Walsh was performed using the interfascial technique, the discovery of supplementary nerve fibers on the anterolateral surface of the prostate promoted the development of the intrafascial technique [31].

2.3.1.3 The Intrafascial Dissection

Potdevin et al. reported a great improvement of potency rate and reduction of the time to return of continence after athermal intrafascial robotic (AIR) approach. Nevertheless, this improved outcome was achieved at the price of higher PSM rates in patients with pT3 disease. Athermal intrafascial robotic approach allows to identify the plane between the prostatic capsule and prostatic fascia at the posterolateral and anterolateral portions of the prostate. Following this plane of dissection maximizes NVB preservation, thus achieving the best potency outcomes [32]. A recent metanalysis compared intrafascial and interfascial dissection. With regard to the functional results, intrafascial dissection had advantages in terms of both continence and potency recovery. In reference to the oncologic results, the intrafascial approach showed lower PSM compared to interfascial dissection [33].

2.3.1.4 The "Veil of Aphrodite"

The "veil of Aphrodite" is a modified nerve-sparing technique. The prostatic fascia is detached from the prostate and remains as a supportive structure over the ipsilateral NVB. After this step, the periprostatic tissue along with the NVBs hangs like a curtain from the pubourethral ligaments. In sequence, the bilateral NVB release (posterolateral) is performed from 5 to 1 o'clock on the right side and from 7 to 11 o'clock on the left side [34]. This technique has shown better functional outcomes which can be explained by the reduced traction injury to the posterolateral NVB during a precise dissection on the lateral surface of the prostate, reducing the neurapraxia of the cavernous nerves.

2.3.2 Direction of Dissection

2.3.2.1 The Retrograde Approach

Patel et al. described their technique of early retrograde release of the NVBs during robotic-assisted radical prostatectomy (RARP) with an athermal technique and minimization of traction. With this approach, the first step is identification of the landmark artery on the lateral aspect of the prostate. Then, a plane is obtained between the artery and the prostate, which is continued posteriorly, and the dissection proceeds in a retrograde manner toward the base of the prostate. The retrograde approach has the advantage of allowing early recognition and release of the NVB from the prostate, before controlling the posterior pedicle [29]. In a comparative study by Ko et al., a retrograde nerve-sparing approach facilitated early recovery of potency compared to the antegrade approach without compromising cancer control [35].

2.3.2.2 The Antegrade Approach

After transection of the vascular pedicles, the direction of the dissection is from the base of the prostate toward the apex. The procedure starts with a gentle upward traction of vas and seminal vesicles in order to reveal the prostatic pedicles. After creating the inferior plane between the Denonvilliers layers, the anterior dissection creates a space between the Denonvilliers' fascia, lateral pelvic fascia, and prostate [36]. Currently, the antegrade approach is a widely used among laparoscopic and robotic surgeons.

2.3.3 Near-Infrared Fluorescence (NIRF) and Indocyanine Green (ICG)

The identification of the landmark artery has a pivotal role in performing a nerve-sparing procedure.

Near-infrared fluorescence surgery and ICG use are simple, promising, and non-invasive techniques that can be helpful to identify anatomical landmarks, thus optimizing NVB preservation. A study by Amara et al. demonstrated that landmark artery and its course were identified in 85% of cases, without increasing the operating time [37].

2.4 Periprostatic Fascial Reconstruction: From the Rocco Stitch to the Total Anatomic Reconstruction

One of the main complaints after radical prostatectomy is urinary incontinence. The knowledge of the mechanism of continence recovery after surgery is complex and may involve both preoperative and surgical cofactors. In the last years, it has been demonstrated that the preservation of the anatomical structures responsible of continence, the nerve-sparing approach, and the periprostatic fascial reconstruction can help reestablish the presurgical state [38, 39].

With regard to periprostatic fascial reconstruction, a wide range of techniques has been described, such as posterior musculofascial reconstruction, anterior reconstruction and periurethral suspension, anatomical (total) pelvic reconstruction, preservation of membranous urethral length (MUL), bladder-neck reconstruction, and combinations [40–43].

2.4.1 Description of Surgical Reconstructive Procedures

2.4.1.1 "Rocco" Stitch (Posterior Reconstruction)

In 2007, Rocco B et al. described the application of the posterior reconstruction technique to transperitoneal laparoscopic radical prostatectomy [40]. This technique has been modified by several authors such as Coughlin et al. who applied the posterior reconstruction of the rhabdosphincter to RARP with some minor technical changes [44]. This reconstruction is performed using two 3-0 poliglecaprone sutures (on RB-1 needles) tied together, with each individual length being 12 cm. Ten knots are placed when tying the sutures to provide a bolster. The free edge of the remaining Denonvilliers' fascia is identified after the prostatectomy and approximated to the posterior aspect of the rhabdosphincter and the posterior median raphe using one arm of the continuous suture.

The second layer of the reconstruction is then performed with the other arm of the suture approximating the posterior lip of the bladder neck (full thickness) and the vesicoprostatic muscle to the posterior urethral edge and to the already reconstructed median raphe [8]. The reconstructive suture should not run too laterally since it may damage the neurovascular bundles running lateral to the urethra. The reconstruction of the posterior musculofascial plate reduces intraoperative bleeding, facilitates the urethrovesical anastomosis, and improves early return of continence within the first 30–45 days after RP [45–47].

2.4.1.2 "Patel" Stitch (Periurethral Suspension Stitch)

Patel et al. were the first to describe this suspension technique in RARP basing on the procedure already reported by Walsh during open radical retropubic prostatectomy [48, 49].

A periurethral retropubic stitch is placed using a 12-in monofilament polyglytone suture on a CT-1 needle. The stitch is placed holding the needle two-thirds of the way back and passed from right to left between the urethra and dorsal venous complex (DVC). Then the stitch is passed through the periosteum on the pubic bone. The stitch is passed again trough the DVC and then through the pubic bone in a figure of eight. The suture is tied. The DVC is typically divided later during the operation, prior to the apical dissection of the prostate and division of the urethra. The suspension stitch is followed by bladder neck dissection and mobilization of the seminal vesicles prior to ligation of the prostatic pedicles [48]. The study by Patel et al. showed that the placement of the suspension stitch during RALP results in a statistically significant shorter interval to recovery of continence and higher continence rates at 3 months after the procedure [48].

2.4.1.3 Anterior Suspension Combined with Posterior Reconstruction

Hurtes et al. in their multicenter randomized study showed that anterior suspension combined with posterior reconstruction is a safe and easy-to-perform technique for improving early continence after robotic-assisted laparoscopic prostatectomy [50]. Anterior suspension was carried out passing the needle from right to left between the urethra and the DVC. The needle was then held backward and passed through the periosteum of the pubic bone, from left to right. The stitch was passed through the DVC and the pubic bone again to ensure support and tied. Anterior reconstruction can also be performed after making the vesicourethral anastomosis [51]. Posterior reconstruction was performed using an absorbable suture passed through the Denonvilliers' fascia, at the posterior wall of the bladder. The suture was then passed through the rhabdosphincter, beneath the posterior part of the urethra. Reconstruction was completed by passing the suture back through Denonvilliers' fascia and the tissue of the rhabdosphincter twice [51].

2.4.1.4 Semicircular Support for the Urethra and Vesicourethral Anastomosis

This technique consists of creating a semicircle of surrounding musculature around the vesicourethral anastomosis without injuring the neurovascular bundles. The fibers of the levator ani muscle, Denonvilliers' fascia, retrotrigonal layer, and median dorsal raphe were used to form the dorsal support for the urethrovesical anastomosis. Suture of the arcus tendineus to the bladder neck served as anterior fixation. Sudent et al. reported better urinary continence results than standard posterior reconstruction, with no negative impact on erectile function, complication rate, and oncologic outcome [52].

2.4.1.5 Total Anatomical Reconstruction (TAR)

The TAR technique showed promising results in the early recovery of urinary continence, as well as watertight anastomosis and a low rate of urine leakage. The posterior reconstruction is performed in a triple layer by using a 3/0 "barbed" suture. To create the first layer, the needle is passed into the cranial portion of the previously sectioned Denonvilliers' fascia and the median raphe and is moved from right to left. The second layer involves the retrotrigonal fascia and the median raphe and is moved from left to right. The third layer involves the bladder neck (excluding the mucosa of the bladder) and the posterior aspect of the rhabdosphincter. After the urethrovesical anastomosis, the muscular fibers of the bladder are sutured to the previously dissected periurethral tissue, which is located between the urethra and the DVC (anterior reconstruction). Using the same suture and returning to the starting point, the visceral layer of the endopelvic fascia and the underlying apron are sutured to the portion of the endopelvic fascia that covers the DVC (recreation of the "pubovesical" ligaments) [53].

2.5 Periprostatic Fascia Preservation

Reduced fascia preservation has been identified as an independent predictor of worse urinary continence and erectile function [21, 54]. However, technique and degree of fascia preservation have changed over time. Walsh and Donker provided the first description of the distribution of neural structure around the prostate indicating the dorsolateral periprostatic tissue as the most important zone to be preserved for postoperative erectile function recovery [21]. However, after the description of significant branches of the pelvic plexus traveling more anteriorly on the prostatic surface [55], a more extensive fascia preservation was shown to be associated to benefit in urinary and sexual outcomes after prostatectomy [56]. This led to the introduction of several technique, such as the veil of Aphrodite technique, i.e., the high anterior and lateral dissection sparing as much periprostatic fascia as possible, introduced by Menon [57]. Likewise, a "high anterior release technique" was described for open radical prostatectomy as well [54]. Following steps in this field aimed toward the preservation of the Retzius space and the anatomical structures within it which represent the anterior bladder attachment (puboprostatic ligaments, dorsal venous complex, anterior detrusor apron, pubourethral ligament, the arcus tendinous, and the accessory pudendal arteries).

Bocciardi's group developed a modification to RARP respecting the whole space of Retzius by approaching the prostate and the bladder neck posteriorly through the rectovesical pouch [58]. The Retzius-sparing approach (RS-RALP) showed superior results about early recovery of continence [59]. The integrity of the anatomical structures that compose the anterior suspensory mechanism prevents the prolapse of the vesicourethral anastomosis [60]. The correlation between the anterior suspension and the improvement of continence outcomes was firstly observed in retropubic open prostatectomy [61]. More recently, Olgin et al. revealed that a higher bladder neck to pubic symphysis ratio (BNPS), meaning a lower placement of the bladder-urethral anastomosis, was associated to worse continence recovery [62]. Further series confirmed BNPS as a risk factor for postoperative incontinence after laparoscopic and robotic RP [63]. In a propensity score matching analysis, Chang et al. compared BNPS after Retzius-sparing and standard RARP. The ratio was significantly lower in the Retzius-sparing group, and early continence within the first week was 73.3% compared to 26.7%, even if no difference was seen at 1 year [64]. Moreover, special considerations deserve to be made about the DVC preservation. Anatomical studies focusing on the topographic anatomy of the urethral sphincter showed that the DVC covers it dorsally and laterally. Therefore, transverse ligation of the DVC can potentially include a significant part of the urethral sphincter, negatively affecting postoperative continence [65]. A recent metanalysis confirmed the advantage on early continence recovery for RS-RALP vs anterior RALP, even though the 12-months continence rate remains similar and there is a higher rate of positive surgical margins for stage T2 tumors after RS-RALP [66]. Despite these results, the steep learning curve for Retzius-sparing prostatectomy still leads many surgeons to perform an anterior approach. More recently, a new surgical technique that combines the advantages of preserving the Retzius space landmarks while using an anterior approach has been described by Tewari's group [67]. This approach has been published as "hood technique" since the periprostatic tissue spared after prostate removal (arcus tendineus, puboprostatic ligament, detrusor apron, DVC, anterior periprostatic fascia, and the underlying fibers of the detrusor muscle) has a parabolic shape. These structures surround and protect the membranous urethra and external sphincter during dissection of the prostate apex and support the anastomosis. Functional data available to date show that the hood technique is associated to early return of continence after surgery, without causing an increase in positive surgical margin rates [67].

Currently, the use of the robotic approach leads to resume also perineal radical prostatectomy [6]. The perineal route has been the first surgical approach to prostatectomy since 1905 [68], but it has been set aside for a long time after the advent of retropubic radical prostatectomy. Either the Xi® and the single-port robotic platforms characteristics facilitate the perineal approach by minimizing arms clashing and enhancing instruments mobility and ergonomics during the critical steps of the procedure [69]. Since the perineal approach does not imply the division of the anterior periprostatic fascia, it is de facto a Retzius-sparing approach which left untouched the anterior suspensory mechanism of the bladder [70]. In the largest available series, recovery of urinary continence occurred in 41% and 91% of the patients immediately and 12 months after robotic perineal radical prostatectomy, respectively [71]. The same group reported normal 12-months erectile function in 77% of men who did not have preoperative erectile dysfunction [71].

2.6 Bladder Neck Preservation

The bladder neck is the anatomic area identified both as the point of bladder outlet and the beginning of the prostatic urethra. It histologically consists of a number of different structures: detrusor muscle, vesical sphincter, and adjacent proximal prostatic tissue [8].

Anteriorly and laterally, there is a contiguity between detrusor fibers and bladder neck, but there is not a contribution of these fibers in the composition of the sphincter. Nevertheless, some fibers of the outer longitudinal detrusor layer, by reaching the pubis, result in the formation of puboprostatic and pubovesical ligaments, a complex also called anterior detrusor apron. It can be useful to preserve the latter as it is well recognized as a continence structure [12, 72].

Posteriorly, some fibers of the outer longitudinal detrusor layer cover the trigone and penetrate the back side of the prostate (posterior detrusor apron), without forming part of the sphincter system but anchoring the bladder in the pelvis.

The vesical trigone is a triangulary shaped area extending from back to front from the ureteral orifices to the urethral opening. Trigone is mainly formed by fibers of the vesical sphincter, which is elliptic shaped, with the urethral opening located in the anterior third of the ellipsis and surrounded by circular smooth muscle fibers [73]. The latter ensures continuous urinary continence and at the same time antegrade ejaculation.

The conservation of several muscular and fibrous structures anchoring the bladder neck to the pubis, the preservation of bladder neck, and the angulation between the bladder neck and urethra after vesicourethral anastomosis represent potentially important vehicles to lead to recovery of continence after radical prostatectomy [67].

Bladder neck-sparing technique is commonly performed to improve postoperative continence, but controversies exist about its real effect on this issue.

In general, it is evident that a suboptimal bladder neck dissection may lead to poor outcomes: On the one hand, in oncological terms, a too distal dissection in an attempt to spare bladder neck can result in positive margins. On the other hand, in functional terms, a too proximal dissection can involve ureters or require a bladder neck reconstruction.

Freire et al. compared oncological and functional data after bladder neck preservation (BNP) technique vs standard technique (ST) [74]. No substantial difference was found about positive margin status. Similarly, continence rates after 2 years were comparable for both techniques. Nevertheless, a considerable earlier recovery of continence (zero pads per day) was significantly higher for BNP vs ST (65.6% vs 26.5% at 4 months), which obviously improves quality of life.

Nyarangi-Dix et al. too, in a prospective, randomized, controlled, single-blind trial, have experienced that BNP during radical prostatectomy is paired with a higher urinary continence rate and better QoL without compromising resection margins [75].

BNP is also associated to a lower risk of bladder neck contracture and lower rates of ureteral injury, so it results in lower rates of reintervention for vesicourethral reanastomosis and ureteral reimplantation. Moreover, a wide dissection of bladder neck entails more operative time for its reconstruction.

2.7 Membranous Urethra Preservation

The membranous urethra is the more distal part of posterior urethra and extends from the prostatic apex to the bulbar urethra. It is made of an intrinsic and an extrinsic component. The first one lies within the wall of membranous urethra and is made of a circular layer of smooth muscle fibers able to maintain tonic contraction, thus resulting in continuous continence. The extrinsic component is made of a layer of striated muscle fibers (elevator muscles of the pelvic floor) in contiguity with membranous urethra posteriorly and laterally, thus forming a sort of "pubourethral sling" that inserts into the perineal body anchored to the posterior surface of the bulbo-membranous urethra. These fibers can contract for only brief periods. In fact, its main role is a voluntary interruption of urinary stream caused by compression of urethra from behind.

The internal sphincter at the bladder neck is not strong enough to maintain continence if the external sphincter is injured, hence the importance of preserving membranous urethra while performing radical prostatectomy, although certain aspects can complicate this task.

The rationale behind membranous urethral lengthening (MUL) technique is that an increased urethral length, which includes a greater amount of smooth muscle and the rhabdosphincter, increases the length of the urethral pressure profile. After dissecting the DVC and showing the prostatic apex and the rhabdosphincter, the striated and smooth muscle fibers are smoothly dissected from the prostatic rhabdosphincter junction toward the membranous urethra. Together with the release of fibrous connections of the prostate at the apex, an additional length of the intra-abdominal urethra is obtained. With this regard, the anatomy of the prostate is variable. Sometimes, the apex of the prostate may overlap the urethral sphincter in several ways. Considerable overlap might render the preservation of the entire urethral sphincter difficult [8]. Depending on the individual apex shape, between 10% and 40% of the functional urethra is covered by parenchymal apex tissue [38].

Schlomm et al. [38] described a full functional-length preservation of the urethral sphincter (FFLU) by performing a tailored preparation of the prostatic apex, respecting the length of the urethral sphincter located into the prostate. These authors described a cranial traction to the prostatic apex resulting in a "sliding effect" allowing the exposure of the posterior aspect of urethra cranially to the colliculus and the external sphincter which can be safely cut to release the apex. In this way, the preservation of membranous urethra becomes apex shape independent [38, 76]. In addition, Schlomm performs a fixation of the sphincter by preserving the pelvic floor and reconstructing the Mueller's ligaments. This combination allows complete early continence rate 1 week after catheter removal of 50.1% compared to

30.9% in case of no FFLU approach [38]. Hamada et al. described a modified technique of maximal urethral length preservation and reported a significantly higher continence rate and a shorter period to pad-free status in men undergoing RALP [77]. After the removal of the prostate, not only the external sphincter is divided but also a number of supporting structures are damaged. The reapproximation of the rhabdosphincter to the Denonvilliers' fascia reestablish the anatomical continuity by fixing the sphincter in its natural position: This technique was first introduced by Rocco. The role of reconstruction of the posterior musculofascial plate in terms of early recovery of continence seems to be encouraging but remains controversial. Nguyen, Coelho, Brien, and Gondo agree on the earlier recovery of urinary continence by using posterior rhabdosphincter reconstruction vs standard technique [39, 40, 78, 79]. In contrast, according to Joshi and Sutherland, posterior rhabdosphincter reconstruction does not offer any advantage for the return of early continence after RARP [80, 81].

2.8 Conclusion

Urinary incontinence and erectile dysfunction represent the most bothersome complications following radical prostatectomy: Up to 15% of patient will suffer from permanent urinary incontinence while higher proportion of patient will be unable to achieve a satisfactory erection long term. Robotic surgery has led to a better access to the pelvis, magnification of the surgical field, and improved surgical dexterity resulting in a significant improvement in these functional outcomes. Specific tips and tricks aiming to a better preservation of the neurovascular bundles and reconstruction and preservation of the bladder neck, urinary sphincter, and periurethral structures have been described by experienced surgeons but the effective impact on potency and continence not infrequently remain controversial.

Acknowledgments The workgroup gratefully acknowledges the contribution of Dr. Giuseppe Papapicco for the pictures included in this chapter.

References

1. Mottet N, van den Bergh RCN, Briers E, et al. EAU-EANM-ESTRO-ESUR-SIOG guidelines on prostate cancer-2020 update. Part 1: screening, diagnosis, and local treatment with curative intent. Eur Urol. 2021;79:243–62.
2. Milsom I, Altman D, Nelson R, Sillén U, Thom D. Epidemiology of urinary (UI) and faecal (FI) incontinence and pelvic organ prolapse (POP). www.ics.org/Publications.
3. Michl UHG, Friedrich MG, Graefen M, Haese A, Heinzer H, Huland H. Prediction of postoperative sexual function after nerve sparing radical retropubic prostatectomy. J Urol. 2006;176:227–31.
4. Walsh PC. Radical prostatectomy for the treatment of localized prostatic carcinoma. Urol Clin North Am. 1980;7:583–91.
5. Costello AJ. Considering the role of radical prostatectomy in 21st century prostate cancer care. Nat Rev Urol. 2020;17:177–88.

6. Minafra P, Carbonara U, Vitarelli A, Lucarelli G, Battaglia M, Ditonno P. Robotic radical perineal prostatectomy: tradition and evolution in the robotic era. Curr Opin Urol. 2021;31:11–7.
7. Ficarra V, Novara G, Artibani W, et al. Retropubic, laparoscopic, and robot-assisted radical prostatectomy: a systematic review and cumulative analysis of comparative studies. Eur Urol. 2009;55:1037–63.
8. Walz J, Epstein JI, Ganzer R, et al. A critical analysis of the current knowledge of surgical anatomy of the prostate related to optimisation of cancer control and preservation of continence and erection in candidates for radical prostatectomy: an update. Eur Urol. 2016;70:301–11.
9. Martini A, Tewari AK. Anatomic robotic prostatectomy: current best practice. Ther Adv Urol. 2019;11:1756287218813789.
10. Steiner MS. The puboprostatic ligament and the male urethral suspensory mechanism: an anatomic study. Urology. 1994;44:530–4.
11. Wimpissinger TF, Tschabitscher M, Feichtinger H, Stackl W. Surgical anatomy of the puboprostatic complex with special reference to radical perineal prostatectomy. BJU Int. 2003;92:681–4.
12. Walz J, Burnett AL, Costello AJ, et al. A critical analysis of the current knowledge of surgical anatomy related to optimization of cancer control and preservation of continence and erection in candidates for radical prostatectomy. Eur Urol. 2010;57:179–92.
13. Raychaudhuri B, Cahill D. Pelvic fasciae in urology. Ann R Coll Surg Engl. 2008;90:633–7.
14. van Ophoven A, Roth S. The anatomy and embryological origins of the fascia of Denonvilliers: a medico-historical debate. J Urol. 1997;157:3–9.
15. Weldon VE, Tavel FR. Potency-sparing radical perineal prostatectomy: anatomy, surgical technique and initial results. J Urol. 1988;140:559–62.
16. Khattar N, Nayyar R, Sood R. Perineal prostatectomy. In: Khanna RV, Bratslavsky G, Stein RJ, editors. Surgical techniques for prostate cancer. New York: Springer; 2015. p. 61–78.
17. Mauroy B, Demondion X, Drizenko A, Goullet E, Bonnal J-L, Biserte J, Abbou C. The inferior hypogastric plexus (pelvic plexus): its importance in neural preservation techniques. Surg Radiol Anat. 2003;25:6–15.
18. Takenaka A, Tewari AK. Anatomical basis for carrying out a state-of-the-art radical prostatectomy. Int J Urol. 2012;19:7–19.
19. Baader B, Herrmann M. Topography of the pelvic autonomic nervous system and its potential impact on surgical intervention in the pelvis. Clin Anat. 2003;16:119–30.
20. Takenaka A, Kawada M, Murakami G, Hisasue S, Tsukamoto T, Fujisawa M. Interindividual variation in distribution of extramural ganglion cells in the male pelvis: a semi-quantitative and immunohistochemical study concerning nerve-sparing pelvic surgery. Eur Urol. 2005;48:46–52; discussion 52.
21. Walsh PC, Donker PJ. Impotence following radical prostatectomy: insight into etiology and prevention. J Urol. 1982;128:492–7.
22. Tewari A, Takenaka A, Mtui E, Horninger W, Peschel R, Bartsch G, Vaughan ED. The proximal neurovascular plate and the tri-zonal neural architecture around the prostate gland: importance in the athermal robotic technique of nerve-sparing prostatectomy. BJU Int. 2006;98:314–23.
23. Costello AJ, Dowdle BW, Namdarian B, Pedersen J, Murphy DG. Immunohistochemical study of the cavernous nerves in the periprostatic region. BJU Int. 2011;107:1210–5.
24. Eichelberg C, Erbersdobler A, Michl U, Schlomm T, Salomon G, Graefen M, Huland H. Nerve distribution along the prostatic capsule. Eur Urol. 2007;51:105–10; discussion 110–111.
25. Steineck G, Bjartell A, Hugosson J, et al. Degree of preservation of the neurovascular bundles during radical prostatectomy and urinary continence 1 year after surgery. Eur Urol. 2015;67:559–68.
26. Avulova S, Zhao Z, Lee D, et al. The effect of nerve sparing status on sexual and urinary function: 3-year results from the CEASAR study. J Urol. 2018;199:1202–9.
27. Axén E, Godtman RA, Bjartell A, et al. Degree of preservation of neurovascular bundles in radical prostatectomy and recurrence of prostate cancer. Eur Urol Open Sci. 2021;30:25–33.
28. Schatloff O, Chauhan S, Sivaraman A, Kameh D, Palmer KJ, Patel VR. Anatomic grading of nerve sparing during robot-assisted radical prostatectomy. Eur Urol. 2012;61:796–802.

29. Kumar A, Patel VR, Panaiyadiyan S, Seetharam Bhat KR, Moschovas MC, Nayak B. Nerve-sparing robot-assisted radical prostatectomy: current perspectives. Asian J Urol. 2021;8:2–13.
30. Kyriazis I, Spinos T, Tsaturyan A, Kallidonis P, Stolzenburg JU, Liatsikos E. Different nerve-sparing techniques during radical prostatectomy and their impact on functional outcomes. Cancers. 2022;14:1601.
31. Stolzenburg J-U, Kallidonis P, Do M, et al. A comparison of outcomes for interfascial and intrafascial nerve-sparing radical prostatectomy. Urology. 2010;76:743–8.
32. Potdevin L, Ercolani M, Jeong J, Kim IY. Functional and oncologic outcomes comparing interfascial and intrafascial nerve sparing in robot-assisted laparoscopic radical prostatectomies. J Endourol. 2009;23:1479–84.
33. Weng H, Zeng X-T, Li S, Meng X-Y, Shi M-J, He D-L, Wang X-H. Intrafascial versus interfascial nerve sparing in radical prostatectomy for localized prostate cancer: a systematic review and meta-analysis. Sci Rep. 2017;7:11454.
34. Kaul S, Savera A, Badani K, Fumo M, Bhandari A, Menon M. Functional outcomes and oncological efficacy of Vattikuti Institute prostatectomy with Veil of Aphrodite nerve-sparing: an analysis of 154 consecutive patients. BJU Int. 2006;97:467–72.
35. Ko YH, Coelho RF, Sivaraman A, Schatloff O, Chauhan S, Abdul-Muhsin HM, Carrion RJV, Palmer KJ, Cheon J, Patel VR. Retrograde versus antegrade nerve sparing during robot-assisted radical prostatectomy: which is better for achieving early functional recovery? Eur Urol. 2013;63:169–77.
36. Carini M, Masieri L, Minervini A, Lapini A, Serni S. Oncological and functional results of antegrade radical retropubic prostatectomy for the treatment of clinically localised prostate cancer. Eur Urol. 2008;53:554–61.
37. Amara N, Al Youssef T, Massa J, Fidjel A, Khoury EE, Patel B, Flais M, Deswarte C. Intraoperative angiography of the neurovascular bundle using indocyanine green and near-infrared fluorescence improves anatomical dissection during robot-assisted radical prostatectomy: initial clinical experience. J Robot Surg. 2022;17:687. https://doi.org/10.1007/s11701-022-01483-w.
38. Schlomm T, Heinzer H, Steuber T, Salomon G, Engel O, Michl U, Haese A, Graefen M, Huland H. Full functional-length urethral sphincter preservation during radical prostatectomy. Eur Urol. 2011;60:320–9.
39. Ficarra V, Novara G, Rosen RC, et al. Systematic review and meta-analysis of studies reporting urinary continence recovery after robot-assisted radical prostatectomy. Eur Urol. 2012;62:405–17.
40. Rocco B, Gregori A, Stener S, Santoro L, Bozzola A, Galli S, Knez R, Scieri F, Scaburri A, Gaboardi F. Posterior reconstruction of the rhabdosphincter allows a rapid recovery of continence after transperitoneal videolaparoscopic radical prostatectomy. Eur Urol. 2007;51:996–1003.
41. Nguyen MM, Kamoi K, Stein RJ, Aron M, Hafron JM, Turna B, Myers RP, Gill IS. Early continence outcomes of posterior musculofascial plate reconstruction during robotic and laparoscopic prostatectomy. BJU Int. 2008;101:1135–9.
42. Coelho RF, Chauhan S, Orvieto MA, Sivaraman A, Palmer KJ, Coughlin G, Patel VR. Influence of modified posterior reconstruction of the rhabdosphincter on early recovery of continence and anastomotic leakage rates after robot-assisted radical prostatectomy. Eur Urol. 2011;59:72–80.
43. Jeong CW, Oh JJ, Jeong SJ, Hong SK, Byun S-S, Choe G, Lee SE. Novel posterior reconstruction technique during robot-assisted laparoscopic prostatectomy: description and comparative outcomes. Int J Urol. 2012;19:683–7.
44. Coughlin G, Dangle PP, Patil NN, Palmer KJ, Woolard J, Jensen C, Patel V. Surgery illustrated—focus on details. Modified posterior reconstruction of the rhabdosphincter: application to robotic-assisted laparoscopic prostatectomy. BJU Int. 2008;102:1482–5.
45. Rocco B, Cozzi G, Spinelli MG, et al. Posterior musculofascial reconstruction after radical prostatectomy: a systematic review of the literature. Eur Urol. 2012;62:779–90.
46. Montorsi F, Wilson TG, Rosen RC, et al. Best practices in robot-assisted radical prostatectomy: recommendations of the Pasadena Consensus Panel. Eur Urol. 2012;62:368–81.

47. Ficarra V, Wiklund PN, Rochat CH, Dasgupta P, Challacombe BJ, Sooriakumaran P, Siemer S, Suardi N, Novara G, Mottrie A. The European Association of Urology Robotic Urology Section (ERUS) survey of robot-assisted radical prostatectomy (RARP). BJU Int. 2013;111:596–603.
48. Patel VR, Coelho RF, Palmer KJ, Rocco B. Periurethral suspension stitch during robot-assisted laparoscopic radical prostatectomy: description of the technique and continence outcomes. Eur Urol. 2009;56:472–8.
49. Walsh PC. Re: Anatomical radical retropubic prostatectomy: detailed description of the surgical technique. J Urol. 2005;173:324.
50. Hurtes X, Rouprêt M, Vaessen C, Pereira H, Faivre d'Arcier B, Cormier L, Bruyère F. Anterior suspension combined with posterior reconstruction during robot-assisted laparoscopic prostatectomy improves early return of urinary continence: a prospective randomized multicentre trial. BJU Int. 2012;110:875–83.
51. Tan G, Srivastava A, Grover S, Peters D, Dorsey P, Scott A, Jhaveri J, Tilki D, Te A, Tewari A. Optimizing vesicourethral anastomosis healing after robot-assisted laparoscopic radical prostatectomy: lessons learned from three techniques in 1900 patients. J Endourol. 2010;24:1975–83.
52. Student V, Vidlar A, Grepl M, Hartmann I, Buresova E, Student V. Advanced reconstruction of vesicourethral support (ARVUS) during robot-assisted radical prostatectomy: one-year functional outcomes in a two-group randomised controlled trial. Eur Urol. 2017;71:822–30.
53. Porpiglia F, Bertolo R, Manfredi M, De Luca S, Checcucci E, Morra I, Passera R, Fiori C. Total anatomical reconstruction during robot-assisted radical prostatectomy: implications on early recovery of urinary continence. Eur Urol. 2016;69:485–95.
54. Nielsen ME, Schaeffer EM, Marschke P, Walsh PC. High anterior release of the levator fascia improves sexual function following open radical retropubic prostatectomy. J Urol. 2008;180:2557–64; discussion 2564.
55. Costello AJ, Brooks M, Cole OJ. Anatomical studies of the neurovascular bundle and cavernosal nerves. BJU Int. 2004;94:1071–6.
56. van der Poel HG, de Blok W, Joshi N, van Muilekom E. Preservation of lateral prostatic fascia is associated with urine continence after robotic-assisted prostatectomy. Eur Urol. 2009;55:892–900.
57. Savera AT, Kaul S, Badani K, Stark AT, Shah NL, Menon M. Robotic radical prostatectomy with the "Veil of Aphrodite" technique: histologic evidence of enhanced nerve sparing. Eur Urol. 2006;49:1065–73; discussion 1073–1074.
58. Galfano A, Ascione A, Grimaldi S, Petralia G, Strada E, Bocciardi AM. A new anatomic approach for robot-assisted laparoscopic prostatectomy: a feasibility study for completely intrafascial surgery. Eur Urol. 2010;58:457–61.
59. Dalela D, Jeong W, Prasad M-A, et al. A pragmatic randomized controlled trial examining the impact of the Retzius-sparing approach on early urinary continence recovery after robot-assisted radical prostatectomy. Eur Urol. 2017;72:677–85.
60. Cui J, Guo H, Li Y, et al. Pelvic floor reconstruction after radical prostatectomy: a systematic review and meta-analysis of different surgical techniques. Sci Rep. 2017;7:AB059. https://doi.org/10.1038/s41598-017-02991-8.
61. Walsh PC, Quinlan DM, Morton RA, Steiner MS. Radical retropubic prostatectomy. Improved anastomosis and urinary continence. Urol Clin North Am. 1990;17:679–84.
62. Olgin G, Alsyouf M, Han D, Li R, Lightfoot M, Smith D, Nicolay L, Ruckle H, Baldwin DD. Postoperative cystogram findings predict incontinence following robot-assisted radical prostatectomy. J Endourol. 2014;28:1460–3.
63. Kageyama S, Yoshida T, Nagasawa M, et al. The location of the bladder neck in postoperative cystography predicts continence convalescence after radical prostatectomy. BMC Urol. 2018;18:52.
64. Chang L-W, Hung S-C, Hu J-C, Chiu K-Y. Retzius-sparing robotic-assisted radical prostatectomy associated with less bladder neck descent and better early continence outcome. Anticancer Res. 2018;38:345–51.

65. Ganzer R, Stolzenburg J-U, Neuhaus J, Weber F, Burger M, Bründl J. Is the striated urethral sphincter at risk by standard suture ligation of the dorsal vascular complex in radical prostatectomy? An anatomic study. Urology. 2014;84:1453–8.
66. Barakat B, Othman H, Gauger U, Wolff I, Hadaschik B, Rehme C. Retzius sparing radical prostatectomy versus robot-assisted radical prostatectomy: which technique is more beneficial for prostate cancer patients (MASTER study)? A systematic review and meta-analysis. Eur Urol Focus. 2022;8:1060–71.
67. Wagaskar VG, Mittal A, Sobotka S, et al. Hood technique for robotic radical prostatectomy-preserving periurethral anatomical structures in the space of Retzius and sparing the pouch of Douglas, enabling early return of continence without compromising surgical margin rates. Eur Urol. 2021;80:213–21.
68. Young HH. The early diagnosis and radical cure of carcinoma of the prostate. Being a study of 40 cases and presentation of a radical operation which was carried out in four cases. 1905. J Urol. 2002;168:914–21.
69. Francavilla S, Veccia A, Dobbs RW, Zattoni F, Vigneswaran HT, Antonelli A, Dal Moro F, Autorino R, Simeone C, Crivellaro S. Radical prostatectomy technique in the robotic evolution: from da Vinci standard to single port—a single surgeon pathway. J Robot Surg. 2021;16:21. https://doi.org/10.1007/s11701-021-01194-8.
70. Carbonara U, Minafra P, Papapicco G, De Rienzo G, Pagliarulo V, Lucarelli G, Vitarelli A, Ditonno P. Xi nerve-sparing robotic radical perineal prostatectomy: European single-center technique and outcomes. Eur Urol Open Sci. 2022;41:55–62.
71. Tuğcu V, Ekşi M, Sahin S, Çolakoğlu Y, Simsek A, Evren İ, İhsan Taşçı A. Robot-assisted radical perineal prostatectomy: a review of 95 cases. BJU Int. 2020;125:573–8.
72. Myers RP. Detrusor apron, associated vascular plexus, and avascular plane: relevance to radical retropubic prostatectomy—anatomic and surgical commentary. Urology. 2002;59:472–9.
73. Dorschner W, Stolzenburg JU, Neuhaus J. Structure and function of the bladder neck. Adv Anat Embryol Cell Biol. 2001;159:III–XII, 1–109.
74. Freire MP, Weinberg AC, Lei Y, Soukup JR, Lipsitz SR, Prasad SM, Korkes F, Lin T, Hu JC. Anatomic bladder neck preservation during robotic-assisted laparoscopic radical prostatectomy: description of technique and outcomes. Eur Urol. 2009;56:972–80.
75. Nyarangi-Dix JN, Radtke JP, Hadaschik B, Pahernik S, Hohenfellner M. Impact of complete bladder neck preservation on urinary continence, quality of life and surgical margins after radical prostatectomy: a randomized, controlled, single blind trial. J Urol. 2013;189:891–8.
76. Laucirica O, Gomez E, Hajianfar R, Vilanova JC, Muniesa M. Complete puborectalis, puboperinealis muscle and urethral rhabdomyosphincter preservation in laparoscopic radical prostatectomy: anatomical landmarks to achieve early urinary continence. Int J Urol. 2020;27:525–36.
77. Hamada A, Razdan S, Etafy MH, Fagin R, Razdan S. Early return of continence in patients undergoing robot-assisted laparoscopic prostatectomy using modified maximal urethral length preservation technique. J Endourol. 2014;28:930–8.
78. Brien JC, Barone B, Fabrizio M, Given R. Posterior reconstruction before vesicourethral anastomosis in patients undergoing robot-assisted laparoscopic prostatectomy leads to earlier return to baseline continence. J Endourol. 2011;25:441–5.
79. Gondo T, Yoshioka K, Hashimoto T, et al. The powerful impact of double-layered posterior rhabdosphincter reconstruction on early recovery of urinary continence after robot-assisted radical prostatectomy. J Endourol. 2012;26:1159–64.
80. Joshi N, de Blok W, van Muilekom E, van der Poel H. Impact of posterior musculofascial reconstruction on early continence after robot-assisted laparoscopic radical prostatectomy: results of a prospective parallel group trial. Eur Urol. 2010;58:84–9.
81. Sutherland DE, Linder B, Guzman AM, Hong M, Frazier HA, Engel JD, Bianco FJ. Posterior rhabdosphincter reconstruction during robotic assisted radical prostatectomy: results from a phase II randomized clinical trial. J Urol. 2011;185:1262–7.

Preserving Urinary and Sexual Dysfunctions After Cystoprostatectomy: Surgical Tips and Tricks

3

Yazan Al Salhi, Riccardo Lombardo, Andrea Fuschi, Manfredi Bruno Sequi, Silvio Scalzo, Fabio Maria Valenzi, Paolo Pietro Suraci, Cosimo De Nunzio, Antonio Carbone, and Antonio Luigi Pastore

3.1 Epidemiology and Etiology

Bladder cancer is the most common tumor of the urogenital system and accounts for 10% of all malignant tumors in men. Overall, 75–85% of patients present with superficial bladder cancer at diagnosis, while 15–25% of cases have infiltrating disease [1].

The most common bladder cancer is transitional cell carcinoma, which accounts for 90% of all bladder cancers. The least frequent histological types are squamous cell carcinoma (5%) and adenocarcinoma (1%). Finally, a tiny percentage of bladder tumors are represented by connective tissue neoplasms, such as rhabdomyosarcoma, leiomyosarcoma, and fibrosarcoma.

Bladder cancer is a tumor with a multifactorial etiology, including oncogenic genes (Ras, p21), tumor suppressor genes (p53 and RB), environmental factors, and hereditary factors as risk factors. However, environmental factors, such as tobacco smoke and occupational exposure to aromatic amines, are the most important in the etiopathogenesis of bladder cancer.

Y. Al Salhi · A. Fuschi · M. B. Sequi · S. Scalzo · F. M. Valenzi
P. P. Suraci · A. Carbone · A. L. Pastore (✉)
Faculty of Pharmacy and Medicine, Department of Medico Surgical Sciences and Biotechnologies, Urology Unit, Sapienza University of Rome, ICOT, Latina, Italy
e-mail: andrea.fuschi@uniroma1.it; antonio.carbone@uniroma1.it; antonioluigi.pastore@uniroma1.it

R. Lombardo · C. De Nunzio
Faculty of Psychology and Medicine, Urology Unit, Sapienza University of Rome, Sant'Andrea Hospital, Rome, Italy
e-mail: cosimo.denunzio@uniroma1.it

G. Lamberti, C. De Nunzio (eds.), *Bladder, Bowel and Sexual Dysfunctions Rehabilitation after Radical Prostatectomy*, Urodynamics, Neurourology and Pelvic Floor Dysfunctions, https://doi.org/10.1007/978-3-031-76341-0_3

3.2 Muscular Invasive Bladder Cancer (MIBC)

Radical cystectomy (RC) represents the "gold standard" for muscle-invasive bladder cancer, recurrent noninvasive bladder cancers, radiation injury, and severe end-stage bladder dysfunction. Cystoprostatectomy involves the complete removal of the bladder, prostate, vas deferens, and seminal vesicles, and contextual urinary diversion is performed [2].

As with other pelvic surgeries, cystoprostatectomy is associated with significant sexual dysfunction in both men and women. Erectile dysfunction (ED) affects 80% of patients who undergo RC with urinary diversion due to injuries to the cavernous nerves situated in the neurovascular bundles (NVB). Direct nerve injury, neuropathy, inflammation and fibrosis, hormonal changes, and ischemia explain ED [3]. Furthermore, even among men who regain some sexual function, their vis erigendi does not permit penetration. Studies have documented low rates of return of erectile function following cystectomy and urinary diversion [4]. In addition to ED, several other factors may also impair sexual function following cystectomy, such as body image alterations significantly associated with non-continent urinary diversions.

The choice of orthotopic neobladder (ONB), ileal conduit, or continent cutaneous urinary diversion is critical and depends on patient- and physician-related factors. The advantages of ONB include improved body image and the ability to have spontaneous voiding without an external appliance [5].

The functional goals of ONBs are to create a reservoir comparable to the native bladder, with adequate low-pressure storage and socially acceptable voiding. Dysfunction in either domain can manifest as urinary incontinence or urinary retention. ONBs achieve respectable continency rates, varying from 70% to 100% during the day, while nighttime continence rates typically drop as low as 50%. Furthermore, continence rates improve with time, with 92% of patients reporting continence improvement 12-month postop [6]. The two most common types of neobladder performed are that of Hautmann [7], which uses approximately 70 cm of ileum, and Studer [8], which uses approximately 60 cm. Both rely on detubularized segments of the bowel that are reconfigured into a spherical shape. Detubularization eliminates unwanted contractions that may increase pressure via peristaltic activity, while the spherical construction allows for increased capacity. One purported reason for the improvement in continence over time is an increased capacity and decreased pressure as the bowel stretches. The median capacity for ileal ONBs typically increases to 500 cc after 1 year, regardless of the technique.

An intact external urinary sphincter is essential in achieving urinary continence. However, even if preserved, the sphincter is under autonomic voluntary control. Nocturnal incontinence occurs from sphincter relaxation in conjunction with the lack of detrusor-sphincter feedback prior to RC [9]. The relationship between pouch capacity, pressure, and sphincter function is evident in the nocturnal setting, where incontinence is more likely to occur in patients with a relaxed sphincter, higher pouch pressures, and more significant residual urine. Detubularization and creating an ONB with adequate volume and pressure are essential in attaining proper reservoir storage for continence. An adequate ONB outlet can be obtained through meticulous apical dissection to provide urethral length and nerve-sparing techniques. Preservation of nerve branches from the pelvic plexus and pelvic branch of the pudendal nerve is known to preserve control of the urinary sphincter and supporting the pelvic floor but also preserves sensation in the membranous urethra. This preservation of sensation explains nerve-sparing procedures' ability to improve daytime and nighttime continence, as some have suggested that leakage of urine into the membranous urethra produces either a reflex or voluntary contraction of the external sphincter. In males, nerve sparing during RC is performed as in radical prostatectomy with preservation of the neurovascular bundles that traverse along the posterolateral plane of the prostate [10]. Additional techniques that have been reported to avoid nerve injury and maintain urethral support during RC include pelvic organ-sparing operations. In men, this includes prostate-sparing RC, and in females, uterine- and vaginal-sparing RC. A recent multicenter study from Europe included 185 patients who, after extensive evaluation to exclude prostate cancer or urothelial cancer at the bladder neck and prostatic urethra, underwent prostate-sparing surgery. After a median of 7.5 years, daytime continence was 95.6%, and nighttime was 70.2%. Emptying failure following ONB construction is a known but uncommon risk of surgery. Definitions of emptying failure vary in the literature and include either a complete inability to void or a need for catheterization due to high PVR. Catheterization rates in males vary from 3.9% to 43%, with rates of catheterization due to complete inability to void ranging from 1.7% to 5.3% of men. The etiology of emptying failure after ONB has been attributed to mechanical obstruction or dysfunctional voiding (defined as a post-void residual (PVR) >100 cc) without signs of obstruction. Mechanical obstruction cases are due to anastomotic strictures, neobladder mucosal protrusion into the urethra, the presence of foreign bodies, and local tumor recurrence. The patients with dysfunctional voiding were managed indefinitely with intermittent catheterization [11].

While the etiology of dysfunctional voiding is less understood and diagnosed only after excluding mechanical obstruction, the mechanism proposed to explain the abovementioned phenomenon is a lack of coordination between sphincter relaxation and abdominal straining. Increased abdominal pressure with voluntary external sphincter relaxation permits urine evacuation in ONB patients. While the physiological reflex arc cannot be achieved due to bladder excision, preserving the pudendal nerve permits the voluntary relaxation of the external sphincter. Other nonobstructive causes of urinary retention include elongation and kinking of the neobladder neck and progressive pouch enlargement with neobladder atony [12].

Several surgical principles in ONB creation ensure adequate emptying. For example, placement of the neourethra in the most dependent portion of the reservoir, prevention of excessive funneling of the neobladder neck, and creation of a small but adequate capacity reservoir have been described, but it is unclear whether these have a significant impact on urinary retention or continence.

Different techniques have been described in order to preserve sexual and urinary function.

These are nerve-sparing RC, supra-ampullar cystectomy, and capsule-sparing, seminal-sparing, and prostate-sparing cystectomy. Prostate and capsule sparing are indicated only in highly selected patients due to the risk of local tumor recurrence.

The patient's general condition should advise the choice of urinary diversion. For example, ureterocutaneousneostomy and ileal conduit are ideal for elderly patients and those with impaired renal function because the bowel segment is short and there is minimal contact time with urine. ONB should instead be the diversion of choice for young patients.

In this chapter, we will discuss the surgical techniques which aim to aid sexual and urinary function.

3.3 Nerve-Sparing Radical Cystectomy

3.3.1 Patient Positioning and Preparation

The patient is placed in a hyperextended supine position, with the umbilicus, legs abducted, and knees flexed over the break. Drapes should be positioned after careful sterile preparations with a povidone-iodine solution of the abdomen, scrotum, and perineum and after the sterile insertion of a Foley catheter. Midline umbilicus-pubic incision extended above the navel is performed, incising the rectus and the transversalis fascia. Open, with a Kittner sponge stick in a blunt manner, the Retzius space and develop the laterovesical spaces to visualize the external iliac vessels. Next, incise the peritoneum, ligate and dissect the median umbilical ligament (urachus), and utilize a Kocher clamp on the urachus for better traction (Fig. 3.1).

3.3.2 Mobilization of Bowel and Exposure

The left colon then should be mobilized, incising the white line of Toldt, exposing the ureters. Next, pack with radiopaque laparotomic towels the small bowel, exposing both the right and left side of the sigmoid colon symmetrically, and place an abdominal retractor.

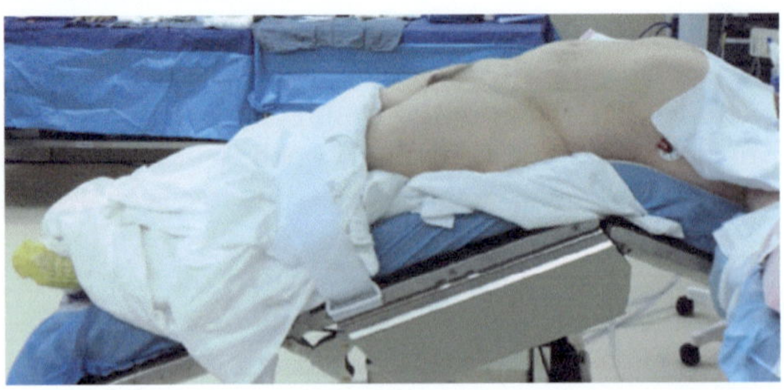

Fig. 3.1 Patient positioning

3.3.3 Ureter Dissection

The peritoneum is incised parallel to the iliac vessels, exposing the ureter that crosses over the mentioned vessels. Place a loop on the ureter to isolate and ligate the superior vesical artery (which runs anteriorly to the ureter). Dissect the ureter at the bladder level after ligating it. Ureters should not be manipulated with any instrumentation to avoid trauma. Bluntly dissect opening a passage from the retroperitoneum to the underside of the sigmoid colon, anteriorly to the sacrum, aorta, and iliac vessels to prevent bleeding. Bring the left ureter to the right side through the McDougal clamp, avoiding its twisting (Fig. 3.2).

3.3.4 Posterior Dissection

Divide the posterior peritoneum sharply under visualization. Establish the dissection plane between the bladder and the anterior rectum and dissect it bluntly with the finger. Expose the seminal vesicles keeping the Denonvilliers' fascia anterior.

Carefully avoid the NVB that runs posterolaterally to the seminal vesicles.

Through GIA stapler, control and divide the posterolateral pedicles, proceeding distally with the dissection, retracting the bladder anteriorly outside the midline incision. Clip the remaining bladder pedicle while bluntly dissecting between the bladder and rectum to further develop the dissection plane.

3.3.5 Anterior Dissection

In order to have optimal visualization of the NVBs and to preserve the nerves running into the membranous urethra, the incision of the endopelvic and periprostatic

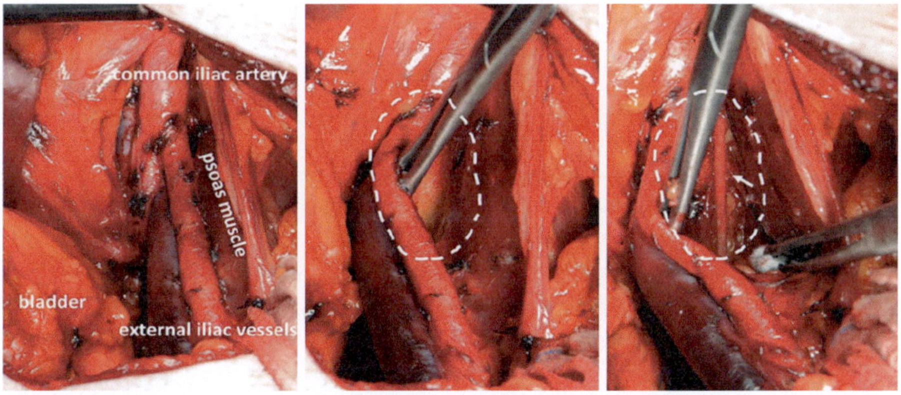

Fig. 3.2 Relationship between the ureters and the iliac vessels

fascia should be approached laterally. Furthermore, the dorsal vein complex should be bunched at the prostate level and not distally to it.

Dorsolateral NVBs are separated laterally from the prostatic capsule. In some cases, the capsule is left in place. Anterior dissection is then completed with the prostatic apex approached laterally. The membranous urethra is dissected sharply with a 15-blade scalpel from the donut-shaped apex to preserve the dorsolateral portion and urethral length. Lymphadenectomy can be performed before the cystectomy or after the piece is removed.

3.3.6 Nerve-Sparing Radical Cystectomy Variation

A variation of NsRC technique was described by Hautmann et al. The technique they describe starts from lymph node dissection. After the dissection of the urachus, a modified lymph node dissection is utilized to preserve the hypogastric plexus sympathetic fibers. These fibers run over the sacral promontory to the hypogastric plexus and the pelvic organs. In their modified template, they preserve the fibers and the lymphatic tissue that overlay the aorta bifurcation and the sacral promontory. The dissection is limited at the level where the ureter crosses the iliac artery proximally and the genitofemoral nerve laterally.

Their group then proceeds with retropubic intrafascial prostatectomy, utilizing a high-release approach offering protection to the NVBs, incising the endopelvic fascia, and bunching the Santorini plexus proximally to the prostate. They then transversally incise the Denonvilliers' fascia for 2–3 cm at the base of the prostate, dissecting the vessels and the seminal vesicles, creating an easily developing cleave plant anterior to the seminal vesicles and dorsal to the trigonal region. Utilizing the catheter's balloon as control, most of the NVBs can be spared and create a dissection plane that reaches the cul-de-sac, preserving the inferior bladder pedicles, performing from then on descending RC. The anterior incision of the peritoneum to the cul-de-sac allows the plane to enter between the SV and the posterior bladder wall, tracing the ureters down to the umbilical and superior vesicle arteries found and clipped [13] (Fig. 3.3).

3.3.7 Seminal-Sparing RC

Seminal-sparing RC differs from NsRC by preserving the seminal vesicles, carefully dissecting ventrolaterally to the SV, and this away from the pelvic plexus.

Different approaches are described.

Ong et al.'s approach begins as a classic RC with a midline incision, with the patient supine in a 30° Trendelenburg position. Bilateral pelvic lymphadenectomy is then performed, followed by the skeletonization of the superior and inferior vesical arteries and their dissection at the level of their emergence from the internal iliac arteries. RC then proceeds with retropubic prostatectomy, incising the endopelvic

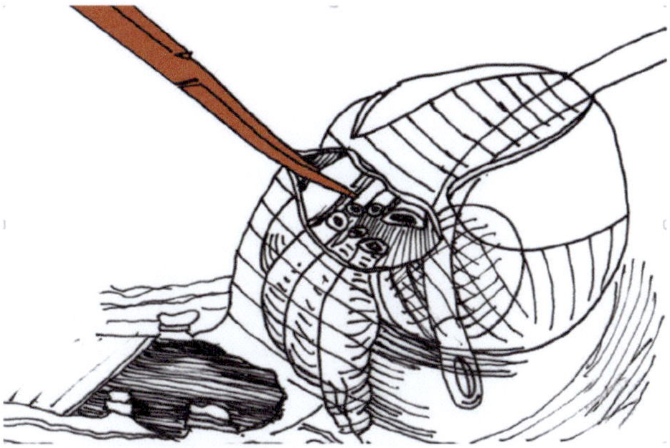

Fig. 3.3 The radical cystectomy is begun as a standard nerve-sparing radical prostatectomy, with high release of the neurovascular bundles. Gentle traction is exerted on the balloon catheter to extrude the vesical neck. Denonvilliers' fascia is opened with a short transverse incision over the ampullae of the vases and the base of the vesicles. After transection of vesicles and ampullae, an easy cleavage plane is developed between the trigone and catheter balloon anteriorly and the vesicles posteriorly until the cul-de-sac has been reached

fascia sharply medially to the tendinous arc. Finally, with a Babcock clamp, the Santorini's plexus is clamped over the prostate apex, exposing the lateral prostate.

Then they identify the ureters and transect them 4 cm cephalad to the bladder. The peritoneum is then transversally incised for 4 cm to access the rectovesical pouch. After identifying the SVs, bluntly dissecting between the SVs and the dorsal bladder wall, a dissection plane is developed toward the dorsomedial pedicle. The dissection must be kept ventrolateral to the seminal vesicle since the pelvic plexus is found dorsolaterally to the seminal vesicle. The dissection then continues caudally toward the vesicoprostatic junction. Next, a lateral incision of the capsule is performed ventrally to the NVBs from the base to the apex. The apex is then approached along the lateral aspect of the capsule, in the direction of the membranous urethra, which is sharply dissected at distally to the verumontanum. Only the capsules covering the NVBs are left in situ.

In this procedure, the three most important steps are dissection ventrally to the SVs, preservation of the NVB at the level of the vesicoprostatic angle, and the incision and cleavage to the dorsolateral prostatic fascia, avoiding damage to the NVBs [14] (Fig. 3.4).

Puppo et al.'s approach differs by sharply dissecting the bladder from the SVs and the deferential ampullae, exposing the ejaculatory ducts. Herein, they don't dissect posterior to these structures, preserving the pelvic plexus, continuing RC with retrograde prostatectomy, in their experience by not transecting the rectourethralis ligament. A cleavage plane is developed over the ligament mentioned above, and the Denonvilliers' fascia, joining the plane previously developed over the SV toward the ejaculatory ducts, preserving even the erigentes nerves of the pelvic plexus [15] (Fig. 3.5).

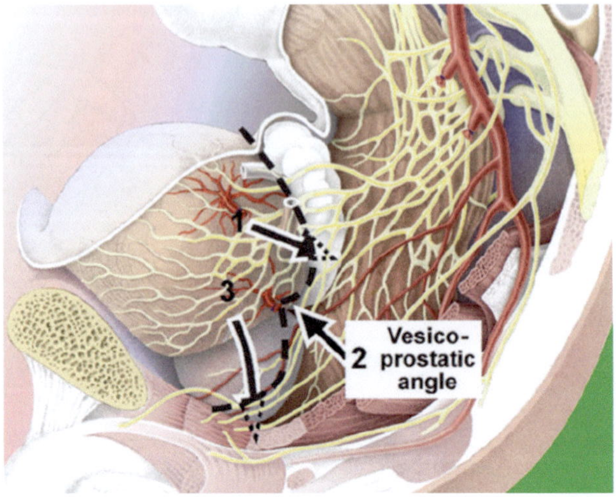

Fig. 3.4 Plane of dissection ventral to seminal vesicle and sequence of dissection

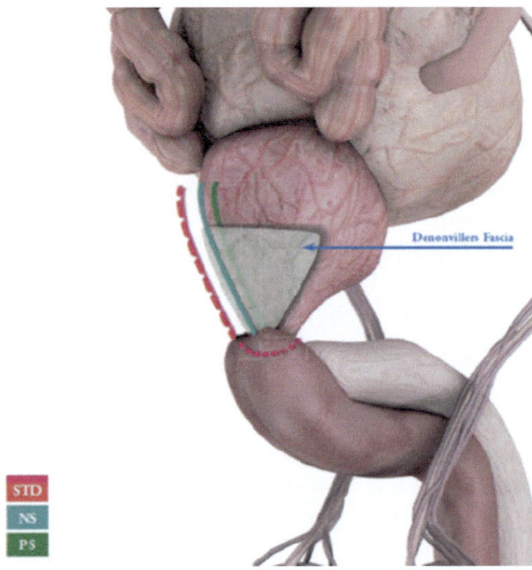

Fig. 3.5 In potency-sparing cystectomy (*PS*, green line), rectourethralis ligament is left untouched and dissection is carried over the anterior leaflet of Denonvilliers' fascia, thus minimizing risk of damaging neurovascular bundles close to the urethra

Salem et al., on the other hand, describe a technique in which the preservation of the SVs is aimed for the preservation of antegrade ejaculation.

In their technique, the vasa deferentia are bilaterally preserved once isolated and dissected at SV level and divided. The dissection is then continued posteriorly to the SVs until the prostatic apex. After ligating the branches of the inferior vesical arteries, the endopelvic fascia is incised. After suturing the dorsal vein complex, the anterior wall of the urethra is incised, and the catheter is extracted and clipped by forceps, creating traction. A posterior incision of the urethra is made, and retrograde Ns prostatectomy is performed. Once transected, the membranous urethra is closed proximally by sutures to ensure anterograde ejaculation. Next, a perineal incision is made to dissect the bulbar urethra. Next, artery forceps are passed on both sides of the bulbar urethra toward the pelvic cavity to cut the ends of the vasa deferentia. Finally, 9-0 Vicryl sutures are used for end-to-side anastomosis between the bulbar urethra and the vas deferens [16].

3.4 Open Orthotopic Neobladder Reconstruction

Ileal reservoirs usually utilize 60 cm of detubularized terminal ileal that can be folded in various ways with the intent of creating a shape similar to the native bladder.

3.4.1 Preparation of the Ileal Segment

A 52 cm of ileum 25 cm proximal to the ileocecal valve is isolated, and the ileocecal valve and the distal 25 cm of the ileum are preserved to reduce malabsorption. The ileal segment is measured along its mesoileum. The distal mesenteric division extends deep into the mesentery to preserve mobility, while the proximal division assures blood supply. Bowel contiguity is restored through standard end-to-end running suture with 4-0 Vicryl. Along the antimesenteric border, the distal portion of the ileum is opened, forming the reservoir of the neobladder.

3.4.2 Ureteroileal Anastomosis

The left ureter is mobilized and transferred retroperitoneally above the inferior mesenteric artery toward the right. Through Nesbit's technique, the proximal ileal segment (afferent segment) is placed medially to the antimesenteric border. The ureters are then spatulated for about 2 cm, and a 4-0 polyglycolic acid suture is then used for a running suture between the spatulated ureter and the seromuscular layer of the ileum. A portion of the ureteral wall is incorporated into the ileal tissue to stabilize the anastomosis. An 8-Fr stent is then placed and secured with 5-0 rapid Vicryl suture that involves both the stent and each side of the ureteral wall. Interrupted sutures can be placed to prevent tension on the anastomosis. Once the stents are placed, the tubular wall is covered with mesenteric fat (Figs. 3.6 and 3.7).

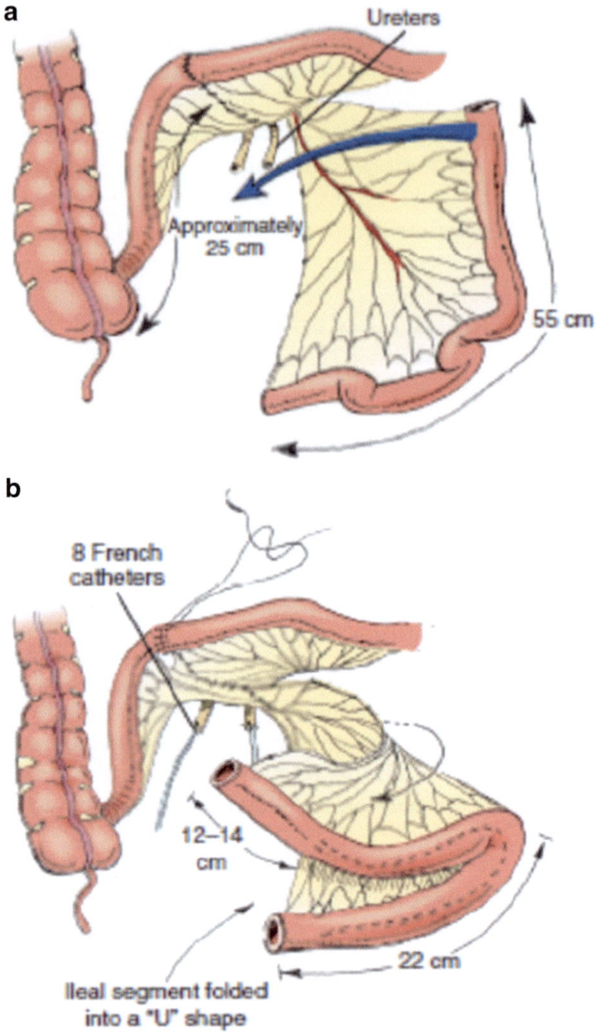

Fig. 3.6 **a**. Ileal segment selection (25 cm from ileal-cecal valve) for neobladder reconfiguration (45 to 55 cm ileal segment). **b**. Ureteral catheters placement (8 Fr, mono J stent) and ileal segment folding to obtain a U shape reconfiguartion

3.4.3 Reconstruction

The distal opened portion of the ileum is folded in a U shape, the medial borders are adapted with a running 2-0 Vicryl suture, and the arch of the U is folded between the two ends to form a low-pressure reservoir, resembling a sphere. At this point, a finger is placed to determine the most dependent portion, and a hole with a 1 cm diameter is excised to facilitate urethral-neobladder anastomosis, avoiding the risk of urethral kinking. An 18-Fr silicone Foley catheter is placed to facilitate the anastomosis. With 2-0 Vicryl suture, the posterior suture passes through the Denonvilliers' fascia and exits at the mucosal edge of the membranous urethra. Two other sutures are placed anterolateral and two anteriorly, including in the Santorini plexus suture and the Denonvilliers' fascia to minimize tension.

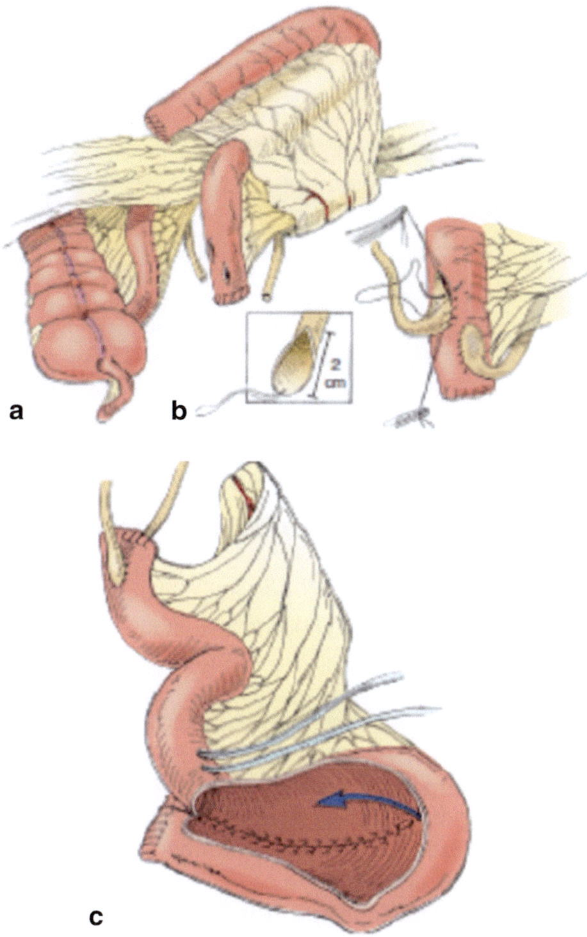

Fig. 3.7 Ureteroileal anastomosis, bowel opening and folding. **a**. Ileal reanastomosis. **b**. Ureteroileal anastomosis. **c**. Neobladder final reconfiguration (folder)

3.4.4 T-Pouch Modification

To preserve the antireflux mechanism, modifications to the T-pouch have been proposed.

The ileum is divided in an afferent end limb long 15 cm, and the distal 4 cm is anchored to the ileal segment at the base of the two adjacent 22 cm segments opened to create the reservoir. In order to reduce the risk of stenosis when the incision on the U portion of the neobladder reaches the afferent ostium, it's extended toward the antimesenteric border, creating a wide flap sutured with 3-0 polyglycolic acid (Fig. 3.8).

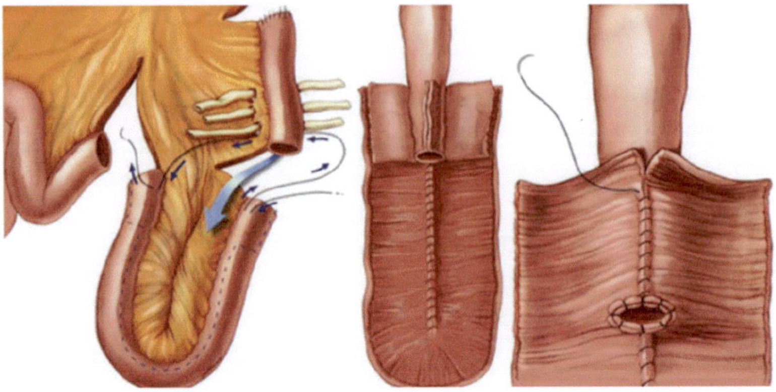

Fig. 3.8 T-pouch modification

3.5 Laparoscopic and Robot-Assisted Radical Cystectomy

Minimal invasive surgery presents advantages such as decreased hospital stay, decreased blood loss, and decreased incidence of complications. The surgical techniques described are the same for laparoscopic RC (LRC) as for robot-assisted RC (RARC).

The required instruments are as follows:

- Monopolar robotic scissors on the first robotic arm
- Maryland bipolar forceps or vessel sealer on the second robotic arm
- ProGrasp forceps on the fourth robotic arm
- Two needle drivers
- Endovascular GIA stapler (optional)
- Hem-o-lok clips (Weck Closure Systems, Research Triangle Park, NC)
- Suction-irrigation device
- Atraumatic grasper

The Da Vinci system is docked between the patient's legs with the robotic arms oriented in a cephalad direction. The assistant is placed on the patient's right. In the case of intracorporeal diversion, the fourth arm is positioned on the patient's right; if extracorporeal diversion is planned, then the fourth arm can be positioned to the surgeon's preference. The control tower is placed left of the patient's left leg adjacent to the instrument table and the scrub nurse. The monitors are located on the top of the control tower and on the opposite side of the assistant.

A sterile catheter is positioned, and the patient is placed in a lithotomy position with the arms tucked.

3.5.1 Port Placement

Six ports are utilized for the operation: a 12 mm camera port, three 8 mm robotic arm ports, and two assistant ports, placed on the opposite side of the fourth robotic arm.

The ports are placed in an inverted V manner, with the camera positioned in the midline, or 3 cm more cephalad in case of neobladder derivations. The two 8 mm ports are placed laterally from the midline (8–9 cm), and the assistant ports are placed laterally and caudally in respect of the robotic port. The fourth robotic arm is then placed laterally to the left port. Finally, through Verres or Hasson technique, pneumoperitoneum is established, the patient is positioned in a 25–30° Trendelenburg position, ports are placed under direct vision, and the robot is docked (Fig. 3.9).

3.5.2 Mobilization of the Sigmoid and Left Colon

A 30° lens is used for pelvic structure visualization. A 0° lens is used after the dissection of the posterior and lateral aspects of the bladder. Identify the urachus and follow the umbilical ligament's peritoneal folds, visualizing the ligaments to the bladder laterally. Incise the peritoneum lateral to the left colon and sigmoid colon on the white line of Toldt, liberating it from the abdominal wall and giving access to the left iliac vessels and ureter.

3.5.3 Development of the Left Paravesical Space

By retracting the medial umbilical ligament medially, the assistant exposes the peritoneum lateral to the ligament and medial to the iliac vessels. The peritoneum is

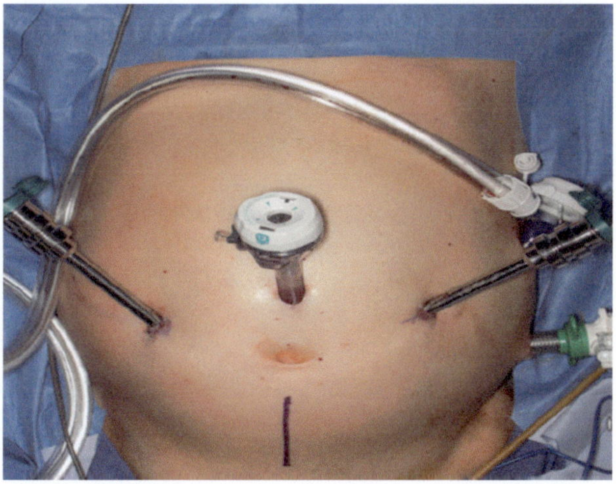

Fig. 3.9 Laparoscopic robot-assisted RC port placement

incised with an incision that extends from the anterior abdominal wall to the bifurcations of the common iliac artery. Use blunt dissection to develop the space. Dividing the vas deferens helps retract the bladder, creating space for lymphadenectomy.

3.5.4 Identification, Mobilization, and Division of the Left Ureter

The ureter is identified at the crossing over the iliac vessels. Its dissection should preserve as much periureteral tissue as possible. The left umbilical artery and/or left superior vesical artery is identified lateral to the insertion of the ureter in the bladder. Clip to gain ureteral length. With a locking clip, clip the ureter, and dissect a portion for the frozen section. The preservation of medial blood supply is critical. The distal ureter can also be tagged with a 2-0 suture.

3.5.4.1 Identification of the Left Iliac Vessels

Medial retraction of the sigmoid colon and bladder gives a visualization of the iliac vessels.

3.5.5 Perform the Left Pelvic Lymphadenectomy

Perform lymphadenectomy with split-and-roll technique utilizing monopolar scissors in the dominant hand and bipolar Maryland forceps. Lift the lymph tissue over the iliac artery with Maryland forceps, bluntly creating a window until identification of the artery wall. Then, Maryland forceps are used to elevate the tissue over the artery, and monopolar dissection is carried out proximally and distally along the vessel shaft. Perform lymphadenectomy, in case of more extended lymphadenectomy, by retracting the vessels medially, a space between them, and the psoas muscles is developed. Care should be taken with the obturated nerve. The split-and-roll technique is highly recommended to avoid injury.

3.5.6 Development of the Right Paravesical Space

After completing the left pelvic lymphadenectomy, attention is directed to the right hemipelvis. First, incise the peritoneum between the medial umbilical ligament and iliac vessels, as done to develop the left paravesical space.

3.5.7 The Right Ureter and Right Pelvic Lymphadenectomy

Due to less colon obstruction, the right ureter is more accessible. Incise the peritoneum that covers the iliac vessels, dissect the ureter, and clip the distal and at the levels of its insertion into the bladder. Perform split-and-roll lymphadenectomy.

After completing the lymphadenectomy, the umbilical and superior vesical arteries are visible. Clip the vessels to avoid using staple loads that risk injuring deeper structures.

3.5.8 Tagging Both Ureters

Using the needle driver, tag the distal end of the ureters with a 2-0 suture on a small half needle to facilitate future retractions for extracorporeal urinary diversion. The suture should be a minimum of 8–10 cm in length.

In the case of intracorporeal urinary diversion construction, clip the ureters creating dilatation that will help with the anastomosis.

3.5.9 Transferring the Left Ureter Through the Sigmoid Mesentery

Transpose the left ureter behind the sigmoid mesentery utilizing the fourth robotic arm. Incise a peritoneum overlying the mesentery, and with a grasper positioned on the right, advance bluntly into the mesentery. Grasp the left ureter and pass it through the mesenteric window.

3.5.10 Tagging the Distal Ileum

If extracorporeal diversion is planned, place a tag on the ileum with 2-0 sutures. The tags should be two; one placed distally to the ileocecal valve and one closer to it to allow for better orientation.

3.5.11 Development of the Prerectal and Posterior Vesical Space

Change the camera lens to a 0° lens for optimal visualization. Incise the peritoneum extending from the posterior bladder to the anterior sigmoid. Develop the prerectal space with blunt dissection. Either the assistant or the fourth arm should retract the bladder anteriorly. Incise the Denonvilliers' fascia for caudal dissection until the rectourethralis muscle.

3.5.12 Lateral Dissection of the Bladder and Control of Vascular Pedicles

Incise the peritoneum lateral to the medial umbilical ligament and divide the vas deferens and dissect sharply between the pelvic wall and bladder (which is retracted away with the ProGrasp on the fourth arm). Clip and divide the obliterated medial umbilical ligaments bilaterally to expose the bladder pedicles. Clip and divide the vessels individually with cold scissors to prevent NVB damage due to monopolar or bipolar energy. The dissection should start from the SV toward the prostate, in proximity to the bladder, to avoid damaging the NVB.

3.5.13 Anterior Dissection, Control of the Dorsal Vein Complex, and Transection of the Urethra

Perform anterior peritoneal incision caudal to the umbilicus, and divide the urachus and medial umbilical ligaments. Mobilize the bladder to access the Retzius space and expose the endopelvic fascia. Incise the fascia and the levator muscles. Divide the puboprostatic ligaments and ligate the DVC with a 3-0 V-Loc suture. Clip the prostatic pedicle and divide it. Separate the NVB down to the prostatic apex. Dissect the urethra circumferentially. Place a 15 mm Hem-o-lok clip on the urethra just distal to the prostatic apex. If the construction of a neobladder is planned, an anterior urethrotomy is performed to preserve a longer length of the urethra just distal to the apex. The posterior urethra is then transected after being clipped with 15 mm Hem-o-lok clips at the level of the verumontanum.

3.5.14 Nerve-Sparing LRC Variation

An interesting variation on Ns minimally invasive RC was proposed by Zhong et al. The rationale for their technique is based on the fact a novel anatomical strategy is required to locate better and preserve erigentes nerves. The novel idea of their technique stems from the accurate dissection of the inferior hypogastric plexus (IHP) before performing pelvic lymphadenectomy.

Once the right ureter is identified, they proceed with the opening of the peritoneum, thus creating a plane between the pre-hypogastric nerve fascia and the peritoneum. The dissection continues caudally toward the rectum where the inferior hypogastric plexus is encountered and dissected laterally to the rectum. On the left side, the retroperitoneal plane is instead developed between the mesentery and the peritoneum on the left sigmoid colon before the IHP dissection.

The subsequent steps differ from standard Ns RC where once the umbilical and superior vesical arteries are dissected and transected, the IHP is under direct visualization, thus easier to spare and preserve during dissection [17].

3.5.15 Seminal Sparing

Similar to open surgery, SV-sparing RC has been described as a viable technique even for minimally invasive surgery. In 2016, Asimakopoulos et al. described their technique for robot-assisted seminal-sparing RC. Port placement and patient positioning are the same for standard RC. Extended pelvic lymph node dissection is then executed, and nodes medial to the ureter are spared to avoid injuries to the hypogastric nerves. The procedure continues with the dissection of the bladder's lateral aspects up to the endopelvic fascia's reflection. Then the rectovesical pouch is opened, and the vas deferens and the SV are exposed. The Denonvilliers' fascia is incised in the area between the SV ampullae, freeing the ventral surfaces of the SV base, preserving the tips and the middle portion and preserving parasympathetic nerve fibers. Next, the NVBs are detached from the lateral prostate-vesicular angle, and the base of the SV is transected. This technique preserves the proximal neuronal network. Intrafascial high-release prostatectomy is then executed. The Denonvilliers' fascia is left in place after lateral dissection of the posterior prostate. Careful dissection of the prostatic apex is necessary since the NVBs run posterolateral to the urethra [18].

3.5.16 Intracorporeal Neobladder

After completing RC and LND, the robotic Da Vinci system is undocked, and the Trendelenburg angle is reduced under laparoscopic vision. Cadiere forceps are deployed on the left arm and fenestrated forceps on the right arm.

3.5.17 Measurement of Bowel Segments

Using either a Penrose drain or an 11 cm suture, 65 cm of the bowel is isolated. A 44 cm will form the reservoir and 16 cm the chimney, and 5 cm will be discarded. Identify the most mobile and dependent part of the ileum to ensure that it reaches the urethra without any tension. Mark this point with a 3-0 V-Loc suture in a Fig. 3.8. This point will become the urethroileal anastomosis (UIA). Measure 11 distal to the UIA toward the ileocecal valve (0-cm point). This point has to be at 15 cm at least from the 0-cm point. Next, measure 11 cm proximally from the UIA (22-cm point). The 0-cm point is where the bowel will be divided, and the 22-cm point will form the apex of the posterior plate (APP). Mark the APP with 2-0 Vicryl suture to identify the cross-folding point of the reservoir. Measure 22 cm proximal to the APP (44-cm point) and mark it with a 2-0 Vicryl suture. This end will form the end part of the reservoir and part of the afferent limb. Next, measure 16 cm (60-cm point) to identify the future afferent limb. The 65-cm point is measured proximally to the afferent limb, and those 5 cm will be discarded. Only the segments selected to restore bowel contiguity should be marked with dyed sutures.

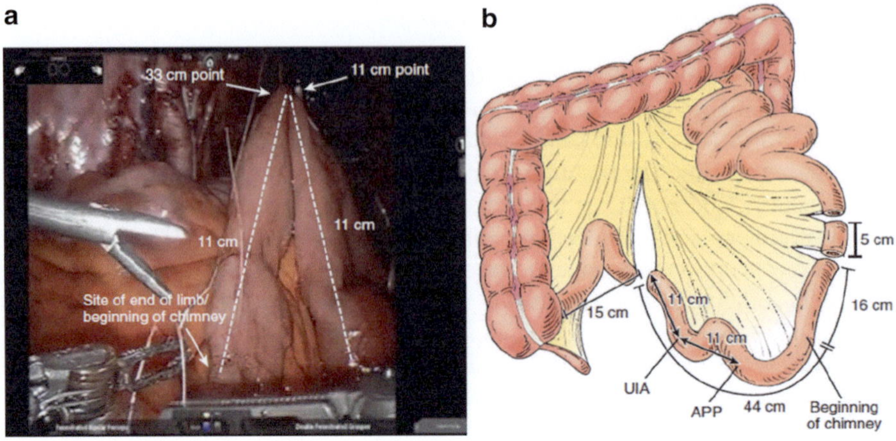

Fig. 3.10 Bowel segment division

3.5.18 Bowel Division and Discard Segment

Divide the bowel at the 0-cm and 60-cm points using a 60-mm stapler. Further staple at 65-cm point with both blue and white (vascular) loads and remove the discarded segment. Once the division is completed, position 2-0 dyed Vicryl sutures to aid side-to-side anastomosis. If any doubts about vascularization exist, for example, indocyanine green can be used with the Firefly system to evaluate the vascularized segments of the bowel better (Fig. 3.10).

3.5.19 Restoration of Bowel Continuity

An opening is made at the antimesenteric ends of the staple line of the two marked ends of the ileum. The assistant inserts a 60 mm stapler with a blue load, and the surgeon guides the ends on the stapler. The stapler is fired twice, and a seromuscular suture is placed to reinforce the anastomosis. The dyed sutures are thus lifted, and the stapler is fired once more on the top side of the anastomosis. A donut is thus created and examined to confirm that the anastomosis is complete.

3.5.20 Bowel Detubularization and Creation of the Posterior Plate

The fourth robotic arm retracts the APP. Enterotomy is performed on the 44-cm point, while a 24-Fr tube is inserted toward the APP. Using monopolar scissors, incise the segment from the 44-cm point toward the 22-cm point. Repeat the incision from the 0-cm point toward the 22-cm point (remember to excise the staple line at the 0-cm point). Open the medial edges of the ileal segments and place four 2-0

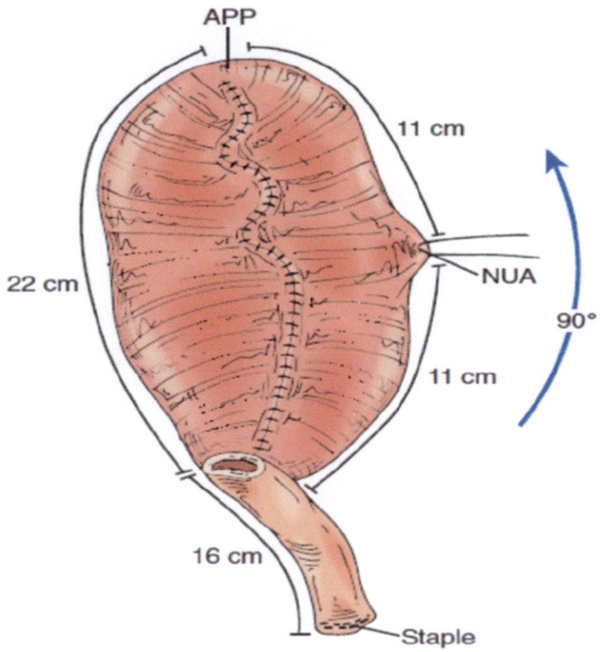

Fig. 3.11 Rotation of the posterior plate. The posterior plate is rotated 90° counterclockwise so that the site of urethroileal anastomosis (11 cm) aligns with the urethra. *APP* apex of posterior plate, *NUA* neobladder-urethral anastomosis

Vicryl sutures to line them up and to create symmetry. From the APP to the chimney, approximate the medial edges with 2-0 V-Loc suture (Fig. 3.11).

3.5.21 Urethra-to-Pouch Anastomosis and Cross-Folding of the Pouch

Rotate the posterior plate to align the 11-cm point with the urethra. Suture the V-Loc suture on the Denonvilliers' fascia. Suture the ileal edge to the posterior aspect of the urethral stump at 6 o'clock with double-armed 3-0 Monocryl suture. Continue the suture up to 12 o'clock. Complete the anastomosis and position a 22-Fr catheter. Use the stay suture at the APP to cross-fold the reservoir at the 0- and 44-cm points. Use 2-0 V-Loc running sutures to close the anterior and posterior lines, creating a sphere.

3.5.22 Ureteral-Afferent Limb Anastomosis

The distal ends of the ureters are trimmed and spatulated, enterotomies are created on the afferent limb, and anastomosis is carried out utilizing 4-0 running Vicryl sutures on RB-1 needles. JJ stents are positioned, and the staple line at the end of the chimney is excluded. To confirm watertightness, infuse about 200 cc of saline and position the definitive catheter with the fourth arm (Fig. 3.12).

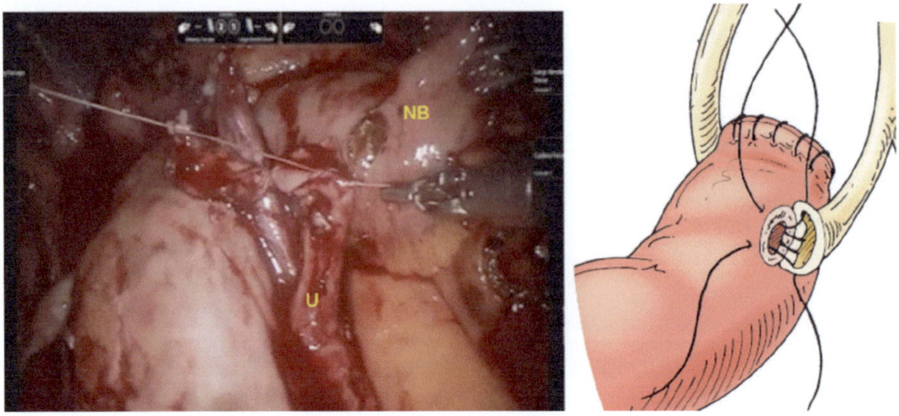

Fig. 3.12 Ureteral-neobladder anastomosis. *U* ureter, *NB* neobladder

3.5.23 Florin Neobladder

Minervini et al. in 2017 described their technique for intracorporeal neobladder construction. First, 50 cm of the ileum, 20 cm from the ileocecal valve, is marked and sectioned, and bowel continuity is restored with base-to-base anastomosis. The urethroileal anastomosis is then performed on a 20-Fr Foley catheter using 3-0 Stratafix suture, folding the ileum in an asymmetrical U shape 20 cm proximally to the anastomosis and 30 cm distally. Detubularization is then performed, and the posterior plate is constructed in an L shape for support. The bladder neck is then confectioned at 12 o'clock from the anastomosis. To create two symmetrical segments, the posterior plate is folded anteriorly 5 cm from the proximal edge of the posterior closure. The ureters are then spatulated, mono J ureteric catheters are inserted, and anastomosis is performed with the 4-0 Monocryl running and interrupted sutures. The anterior plate is closed with an inverted V shape suture with V-Lox 3-0 suture, and the stents are passed through the plate. Finally, the neobladder is filled with saline to check for watertightness [19].

References

1. Saginala K, Barsouk A, Aluru JS, Rawla P, Padala SA, Barsouk A. Epidemiology of bladder cancer. Med Sci (Basel). 2020;8(1):15–21.
2. Modh RA, Mulhall JP, Gilbert SM. Sexual dysfunction after cystectomy and urinary diversion. Nat Rev Urol. 2014;11(8):445–53. https://doi.org/10.1038/nrurol.2014.151.
3. Stenzl A. Pelvic neuroanatomy and recovery of potency. Eur Urol. 2009;55(2):284–6. https://doi.org/10.1016/j.eururo.2008.11.003.
4. Zippe CD, Raina R, Massanyi EZ, Agarwal A, Jones JS, Ulchaker J, Klein EA. Sexual function after male radical cystectomy in a sexually active population. Urology. 2004;64(4):682–5; discussion 685–6. https://doi.org/10.1016/j.urology.2004.05.056.

5. Cerruto MA, D'Elia C, Siracusano S, Gedeshi X, Mariotto A, Iafrate M, Niero M, Lonardi C, Bassi P, Belgrano E, Imbimbo C, Racioppi M, Talamini R, Ciciliato S, Toffoli L, Rizzo M, Visalli F, Verze P, Artibani W. Systematic review and meta-analysis of non RCT's on health related quality of life after radical cystectomy using validated questionnaires: better results with orthotopic neobladder versus ileal conduit. Eur J Surg Oncol. 2016;42(3):343–60. https://doi.org/10.1016/j.ejso.2015.10.001.
6. Clifford TG, Shah SH, Bazargani ST, Miranda G, Cai J, Wayne K, Djaladat H, Schuckman AK, Daneshmand S. Prospective evaluation of continence following radical cystectomy and orthotopic urinary diversion using a validated questionnaire. J Urol. 2016;196(6):1685–91. https://doi.org/10.1016/j.juro.2016.05.093.
7. Hautmann RE, de Petriconi R, Gottfried HW, Kleinschmidt K, Mattes R, Paiss T. The ileal neobladder: complications and functional results in 363 patients after 11 years of followup. J Urol. 1999;161(2):422–7; discussion 427–8. https://doi.org/10.1016/s0022-5347(01)61909-8.
8. Studer UE, Burkhard FC, Schumacher M, Kessler TM, Thoeny H, Fleischmann A, Thalmann GN. Twenty years experience with an ileal orthotopic low pressure bladder substitute—lessons to be learned. J Urol. 2006;176(1):161–6. https://doi.org/10.1016/S0022-5347(06)00573-8.
9. El Bahnasawy MS, Osman Y, Gomha MA, Shaaban AA, Ashamallah A, Ghoneim MA. Nocturnal enuresis in men with an orthotopic ileal reservoir: urodynamic evaluation. J Urol. 2000;164(1):10–3. https://doi.org/10.1097/00005392-200007000-00003.
10. Voskuilen CS, Fransen van de Putte EE, Pérez-Reggeti JI, van Werkhoven E, Mertens LS, van Rhijn BWG, Saad M, Bex A, Cathelineau X, van der Poel HG, Horenblas S, Sanchez-Salas R, Meijer RP. Prostate sparing cystectomy for bladder cancer: a two-center study. Eur J Surg Oncol. 2018;44(9):1446–52. https://doi.org/10.1016/j.ejso.2018.05.032.
11. Simon J, Bartsch G Jr, Küfer R, Gschwend JE, Volkmer BG, Hautmann RE. Neobladder emptying failure in males: incidence, etiology and therapeutic options. J Urol. 2006;176(4 Pt 1):1468–72; discussion 1472. https://doi.org/10.1016/j.juro.2006.06.048.
12. Porru D, Madeddu G, Campus G, Montisci I, Caddemi G, Scarpa RM, Usai E. Urodynamic analysis of voiding dysfunction in orthotopic ileal neobladder. World J Urol. 1999;17(5):285–9. https://doi.org/10.1007/s003450050147.
13. Hautmann RE, Hautmann O, Volkmer BG, Hautmann S. Nerve-sparing radical cystectomy: a new technique. Eur Urol Suppl. 2010;9(3):428–32. ISSN 1569–9056.
14. Ong CH, Schmitt M, Thalmann GN, Studer UE. Individualized seminal vesicle sparing cystoprostatectomy combined with ileal orthotopic bladder substitution achieves good functional results. J Urol. 2010;183(4):1337–41. https://doi.org/10.1016/j.juro.2009.12.017.
15. Puppo P, Introini C, Bertolotto F, Naselli A. Potency preserving cystectomy with intrafascial prostatectomy for high risk superficial bladder cancer. J Urol. 2008;179(5):1727–32; discussion 1732. https://doi.org/10.1016/j.juro.2008.01.046.
16. Salem HK. Radical cystectomy with preservation of sexual function and fertility in patients with transitional cell carcinoma of the bladder: new technique. Int J Urol. 2007;14(4):294–8; discussion 299. https://doi.org/10.1111/j.1442-2042.2007.01607.x.
17. Zhong P, Wu G, Li H, Hu X, Wu B, Guo Z, Zhuo Y, Li X, Lai C. Nerve-sparing laparoscopic cystoprostatectomy based on inferior hypogastric plexus dissection: our initial experience. Urol Int. 2023;107(1):87–95. https://doi.org/10.1159/000524006.
18. Asimakopoulos AD, Campagna A, Gakis G, Corona Montes VE, Piechaud T, Hoepffner JL, Mugnier C, Gaston R. Nerve sparing, robot-assisted radical cystectomy with intracorporeal bladder substitution in the male. J Urol. 2016;196(5):1549–57. https://doi.org/10.1016/j.juro.2016.04.114.
19. Minervini A, Vanacore D, Vittori G, Milanesi M, Tuccio A, Siena G, Campi R, Mari A, Gavazzi A, Carini M. Florence robotic intracorporeal neobladder (FloRIN): a new reconfiguration strategy developed following the IDEAL guidelines. BJU Int. 2018;121(2):313–7. https://doi.org/10.1111/bju.14077.

Bladder, Bowel, and Sexual Dysfunctions Rehabilitation After Radical Prostatectomy: Surgery and Rehabilitation Against Disability

4

Umberto Anceschi, Rocco Simone Flammia, Francesco Prata, Flavia Proietti, Leslie Claire Licari, Eugenio Bologna, Costantino Leonardo, and Giuseppe Simone

4.1 Introduction

Irrespective of the surgical approach considered, radical prostatectomy (RP) represents the cornerstone treatment for patients with localized prostate cancer ≤75 years old [1, 2]. Nowadays, despite advances in preserving pelvic anatomy and a wider availability of different robotic platforms, the overall incidence of post RP bladder, bowel, and sexual dysfunction continues to rise due to the increasing numbers of RP performed worldwide [3, 4].

The prompt identification as the proper management of these specific complications may lead to a quicker recovery after surgery and to a significantly improved quality of life [5]. This chapter focuses on the etiology, evaluation, and management of bladder, bowel, and sexual dysfunction after RP, summarizing current evidence from diagnosis to the best surgical management. A brief discussion of available techniques as their outcomes are also described in this section.

U. Anceschi (✉) · R. S. Flammia · C. Leonardo · G. Simone · F. Proietti
Department of Urology, IRCCS "Regina Elena" National Cancer Institute, Rome, Italy

F. Prata
Department of Urology, Fondazione Policlinico Universitario Campus Bio-Medico, Rome, Italy

L. C. Licari · E. Bologna
Urology Unit, Department of Maternal and Child Health and Urological Sciences, "Sapienza" University of Rome, Rome, Italy

G. Lamberti, C. De Nunzio (eds.), *Bladder, Bowel and Sexual Dysfunctions Rehabilitation after Radical Prostatectomy*, Urodynamics, Neurourology and Pelvic Floor Dysfunctions, https://doi.org/10.1007/978-3-031-76341-0_4

4.2 Anatomical Considerations

"Urinary continence equation" simply requires the pressure in the urethra to exceed that in the bladder [6, 7]. Urethral pressure in men is controlled by multiple mechanisms that include circumferential smooth muscle of intraprostatic urethra and bladder neck, striated pelvic floor muscles, and coaptation of mucosal walls plus the urethral vasculature.

Although described as a sheetlike muscular "urogenital diaphragm," there are multiple muscles involved to constrict the urethra [8]. The striated urethral sphincter (rhabdosphincter/external urethral sphincter) lies at the inferior end of the prostate and generates the greatest urethral pressure of the striated muscles.

Despite not usually considered during descriptions of continence control in men, the levator ani and bulbocavernosus (bulbospongiosus muscle) play a role in constriction of the urethra [9]. The levator ani has three main parts: puborectalis, pubovisceralis, and iliococcygeus. It supports and elevates the urethra via its attachments to striated urethral sphincter [10]. Bulbocavernosus compresses the bulb of penis to constrict the urethra distal to the striated urethral sphincter and in the opposite direction to striated urethral sphincter to assist continence.

4.3 What Happens to the Pelvic Floor After Radical Prostatectomy?

Prostate gland removal causes a multiple trauma to key elements of the continence mechanism [11]. First, RP removes the proximal prostatic urethra including the surrounding smooth muscle. Second, the variability in bladder neck removal or disruption can lead to an improper funneling effect. Third, RP causes potential removal, damage, and scarring of striated urethral sphincter and to its neurovascular supply. Fourth, there is an invaluable disruption of the supporting pelvic connective tissue and ligaments. Fifth, there is a modified detrusor contractility that may be secondary to trauma of the bladder during surgery. Sixth, postoperative stricture/scarring of the vesicourethral anastomosis directly impact urinary flow, also reducing elasticity and urethral closure. Finally, several preoperative anatomical features may also impact final outcomes (e.g., larger prostate size or shorter membranous urethral length) [12].

Among potential mechanisms for incontinence, current literature identifies "sphincter insufficiency" (ISD) as the leading cause (40–88%) [13]. The other common explanations for incontinence are detrusor overactivity (13–67%), but rarely as a sole cause of incontinence, and bladder neck improper funneling. Taken together, these data highlight treatment may be most effective if the striated urethral sphincter is the focus of treatment, whenever possible [14, 15].

4.4 Bladder Dysfunctions After Radical Prostatectomy: An Overview

The major complication of RP remains urinary incontinence, which has significant implications on the patient's quality of life (QoL), and it affects the patient's physical activity and social well-being. Post-prostatectomy urinary incontinence (PPUI) has been reported in 4–69% [16]. Current definitions of "continence" vary from no leakage at all, no pads but loss of a few drops of urine, or use of one safety pad per day, while severe incontinence is often defined as total incontinence or frequent urinary leak and occurs in approximately 8.4% of patients [17]. PPUI represents a multifactorial condition, and it may vary depending on patient characteristics, preoperative continence status, sphincteric competence, pre- and postoperative detrusor function, and surgical factors. In the post-prostatectomy setting, various types of incontinence (stress vs. overflow) or bladder dysfunction may play a role, including poor bladder compliance (PBC) [18]. Overflow incontinence may be secondary to bladder neck contracture or detrusor hypo-contractility. Evaluation should include a deep assessment of medical history and physical along with validated questionnaires to assess symptoms and impact on QoL. Voiding diaries can be useful during this time to document bladder capacity, while bladder ultrasound scans can evaluate emptying. Prior to any planned surgical treatments, patients should undergo urodynamic evaluation (UDS) as well as cystourethroscopy. Additionally, before any intervention is pursued, it is paramount for patients to understand that PPUI can take up to 12 months to resolve without treatment. ISD represents the most important and most common contributing factor to PPUI; however, detrusor overactivity (DO), detrusor underactivity (DU), and PBC commonly occur with ISD or alone and they are all important factors influencing PPUI [19].

Performing UDS allows the clinician to assess, treat, and counsel patient with concurrent bladder dysfunction. If severe bladder dysfunction is identified, its potential complications may be avoided. This can lead to improved quality of life and prevention of complications especially when concurrent treatments of bladder dysfunction may potentially compromise each other [20].

4.5 Detrusor Hyperactivity/Overactivity (DO) After RP

Whether PPUI may result from ISD which is primarily due to injury to the rhabdosphincter during the apical dissection and denervation of the neurovascular bundles during RP, other bladder dysfunction, such as DO, DU, and PBC can be present before RP or may arise after surgery [21].

Mobilization of the bladder during RP can result in partial autonomic and somatic decentralization as well as inflammation, infection, bladder wall alterations, and hypoxia. Preoperative DO can be due to bladder outlet obstruction (BOO) from an enlarged prostate while "de novo" DO may be secondary to BOO from bladder neck contracture or urethral strictures. Several authors suggested that DO may result from urethral afferent activity when urinary incontinence is present [21, 22]. This rationale represents the basis for the reversibility of bladder dysfunction when SUI is successfully treated. Denervation injury to the bladder is the main effect of DU. In analogy to impaired bladder compliance, pelvic surgery such as RP with or without adjuvant radiation therapy can result in bladder fibrosis and contracture, invalidating bladder compliance [23].

DO has been reported to occur at varying rates after RP ranging between 2% and 63%. However, several authors reported that in patients with PPI, only 2% had clinically significant DO [15, 24]. Similarly, the incidence of DO as the primary cause of PPI after RP accounts only for 3.3%. Several authors reported an increased rate of DO in 63% with PPI 8–24 months post nerve-sparing RP [25]. Undoubtedly, DO frequently occurs with other bladder dysfunction post RP, primarily sphincter dysfunction. However, RP can affect preexisting DO in different ways, despite UDS is not routinely performed before surgery. In patients with established preoperative DO, RP does not seem to alter maximum DO pressures. Moreover, several studies showed that DO can improve after RP [26, 27]. According to current literature, preoperative DO rate before RP ranges between 26% and 61%. After 3 years follow-up, the post RP DO rate was found dropped to 17–56%, some of which represent a new-onset condition [28]. Thus, the natural progression of DO post RP can be extremely variable. Some patients with preexisting DO may report a significant improvement after surgery while others may remain stable. Finally, a late onset of DO after RP may also affect a minority of patients (6–12%) [29]. The implications of concomitant DO in men with stress urinary incontinence are noteworthy [30]. For instance, men with DO appear to have worse continence outcomes after a retroluminal trans-obturator sling surgery. Conversely, the presence of DO does not seem to worsen the continence outcome post AUS (artificial urethral sphincter) surgery. However, new-onset or persistent DO-related symptoms occur commonly post AUS surgery and patient needs to be counseled about this medical condition [29].

As a general recommendation, DO should be treated as first step of any clinical/surgical algorithm considered [31]. This will have the effect of reducing the overall PPI and may reveal the real burden of intrinsic sphincter deficiency on PPI [32]. By obtaining a complete recovery from DO, PPI may improve to the point where the patient may not need their incontinence treated or even be treatable by changing the surgical paradigm (with a male sling rather than an AUS). The management of DO related to PPI is determined by its severity and by the presence of ISD, DU, and poor bladder compliance (PBC) [19]. A complete clinical assessment should comprise urinalysis, urine culture, 24-h pad weight, total number of pads, post-void residual volume (PVR), and urodynamic testing. The subjective impact of PPUI may be also assessed with validated questionnaires such as the international consultation on incontinence (ICIQ)—overactive bladder questionnaires [33].

Briefly, the four main treatments currently available for DO are similar to patients affected by LUTS, such as:

(a) Behavioral therapy (bladder training, biofeedback, pelvic floor muscle therapy (PFMT), fluid intake restriction)
(b) Pharmacologic therapy (anticholinergic and β3 agonists)
(c) Invasive treatments (intravesical botulinum toxin (Botox®), sacral neuromodulation (SNM))
(d) Surgery (urinary diversion, cystoplasty)

Data reporting on the use of anticholinergic medications after RP remain scanty despite several authors demonstrated that these medications significantly decreased pad score in patient with DO prior to AUS insertion [34]. Selective β3 agonist showed similar efficacy to anticholinergics but with less side effects that may benefit patients with PPUI-DO [35]. Unfortunately, there is no data reported of their use in the post RP population [36].

Invasive treatments may include intravesical Botox® injection, SNM, and, at last chance, urinary diversion. Intravesical Botox® after RP has an efficacy rate of 30–86% limited by its short-lasting benefit and high rate of retreatment, respectively [37]. However, the risk of urinary retention (about 5%) remains clinically relevant as the patient may be seldom required to perform clean intermittent self-catheterization (CISC). Intravesical Botox may represent an unattractive treatment whenever AUS is planned as repeated cystoscopy or CISC may potentially increase the risk of a cuff erosion [38]. Alternatively, SNM may be considered as an alternative to intravesical Botox® on a theoretical basis. According to current literature, there are relatively few data about SNM in post RP population despite it has a described success rate ranging between 53% and 80% [39]. SNM does not usually cause urinary retention and may extend the treatment to other forms of bladder dysfunction found in association with DO, in particular DU, with recovery rates ranging from 66.7% to 87.4%. Thus, whenever applicable, SNM represents a valid alternative to intravesical Botox® in treating DO post RP. Finally, for severe refractory DO post RP, continued pad use or major open surgery may be the only options remaining. Augmentation cystoplasty is associated with higher rates of CISC (75%) and is not recommended as this may increase the risk of device urethral erosion [40]. Considering a urinary diversion remains another viable option, particularly in patients who might be deemed unsuitable for reconstructive bladder surgery. However, all these challenging treatments must be exhaustively discussed with the patient and contemplated as a final proposal.

4.6 Detrusor Underactivity (DU) After RP

According to ICS guidelines, DU represents "a contraction of reduced strength and/or duration, resulting in prolonged bladder emptying and/or failure to achieve complete bladder emptying within a normal time span" [41].

While a small number of patients have preexisting DU before RP, several patients may develop this condition, mainly because of denervation injury during RP [42]. It has been postulated that minimally invasive surgery has a higher risk of causing DU as it involves a posterior approach to the dissection of the seminal vesicles during antegrade RP where the pelvic nerves are situated. Conversely, during open RP, dissection is performed closer to the seminal vesicles due to traction on the prostate, sparing nerves at the base of the bladder [43]. In the general population, the prevalence of DU is about 9–23% in men less than 50 years, increasing to about 48% in men older than 70 years. The incidence of post RP DU appears to be common ranging between 29% and 61% of patients, of which 47% should be considered as new onset.

Available studies reporting the incidence of DU post RP show major limitations. Firstly, there is no consensus on which urodynamic methodology should be used to identify DU in patients after RP as UDS testing is not routinely performed in this setting. Described methods include the Bladder Contractility Index (BCI), the presence of abdominal straining during voiding and heterogeneous urodynamic cutoffs such as $P_{det}Q_{max} < 20$ cmH_2O or a $Q_{max} < 15$ mL/s [44].

$P_{det}Q_{max}$ in men with ISD may appear decreased due to reduced urethral resistance, and current formulas based on this rationale may be unreliable to diagnose DU. Isometric detrusor contraction pressure (Piso) may represent an alternative metric to diagnose DU. Interestingly, this parameter is measured by gently occluding the penile urethra during voiding, with a Piso of <50 cmH_2O being indicative of DU [45].

Since all available studies did not compare preoperative with postoperative urodynamics findings, the true effect of RP on detrusor contractility may not be currently estimated [46]. Men with DU often void with abdominal straining due to insufficient detrusor strength. However, this may represent a learned behavior as patients with decreased sphincteric resistance may find it easier and faster to void by straining [47].

Therefore, some concern still exists in placing a male sling to treat SUI in men with DU as the sling is designed to create a fixed resistance and may cause urinary retention despite the presence of DU may represent a relative contraindication to its positioning [48].

Regarding the choice of male sling in DU patients, the retroluminal trans-obturator sling offers an advantage over the more compressive quadratic sling. The trans-obturator sling acts by relocating the bulbar urethra and causes minimal compression, whereas the compressive quadratic Virtue is typically tensioned to a pressure of 60 cmH_2O. Thus, DU patients may not be able to generate this pressure and may not potentially be able to void [49].

Conversely, placing an AUS in patients with DU or who are Valsalva voiders post RP appears to be safer and mor effective. The cuff is cycled open with relief of obstruction during voiding. Several series showed no increased risk of raised post-void residual (PVR) or urinary retention post AUS in the setting of DU patients. As DU can present with both voiding and storage symptoms, patients still must be counseled post SUI surgery about the possibility of persistence of common DU symptoms such as urgency, weak stream, straining to void, and nocturia [50].

If a patient can empty his bladder during voiding after SUI surgery, he can be advised to continue to perform an interrupted voiding or use abdominal straining. If there is a decreased bladder storage feeling, the patient may consider a timed voiding. In patients affected by DU before RP or in those with a contractile bladder who are not able to empty the bladder even with abdominal straining, it should be advised they may have to continue or start doing CISC even after PPUI corrective surgery [51].

On the other hand, it is not advisable to perform CISC through a urethral AUS cuff due to the high risk of erosion. Additionally, a bladder neck AUS cuff is also not recommended as it is considered technically difficult and risky in patients where the anastomotic area after RP may be scarred.

In this setting, an adjustable trans-obturator male sling may be considered despite the lack of published data [52]. Compared to AUS which circumferentially compresses the urethra, this device surrounds the bulbar urethra dorsally, leaving the ventral and lateral blood supply intact. The bulbospongiosus muscle is also left intact by acting as an additional protective layer between the device and the urethra [53]. According to current literature, the risk of erosion in this setting appears negligible [54].

Finally, SNM represents a feasible option also in patients with DU, providing a significant increase in voided volume as a significant decrease in mean PVR after SNM treatment. In the general population, SNM placement in DU represents an established surgical option with satisfactory success rates. However, there are currently no published data on SNM in patients after RP [55]. SNM may be theoretically effective also in patients with mixed PPUI. If DU can be successfully treated with SNM first, it may obviate the need for CISC and simplify the subsequent treatment of SUI [56].

4.7 Impaired Bladder Compliance (PBC) After RP

Bladder compliance is calculated by dividing the volume change (ΔV) by the change in detrusor pressure (ΔP_{det}) at a determined filling volume (mL/cmH_2O) during UDS. ICS guidelines recommend two standard points for determination of compliance: firstly, the detrusor pressure at the start of bladder filling and secondly, the detrusor pressure at cystometric capacity or before the start of any detrusor contraction [57].

Poor bladder compliance (PBC) is defined as significant increases in P_{det} with small increments in bladder volume and may lead to incontinence or damage to the upper urinary tract. To date, several definitions on bladder pressure thresholds have been attempted for PBC ranging between $<10\ mL/cmH_2O$ and $<20\ mL/cmH_2O$ [58].

Only few studies have examined PBC in patients with PPUI. Considering the lack of consensus on PBC identification criteria, its incidence stands on 5–28% in the post-RP setting [59]. Despite the high variability reported, urologists should be advised that impaired compliance in severely incontinent patients with ISD may be common but artifactual due to supraphysiologic filling of chronically under-filled bladders during urodynamics and it may be overestimated [60].

Impaired or PBC can be managed with observation and conservative measures such as timed voiding, anticholinergics medications, beta-3-agonists, or intravesical

Botox®. Anticholinergics medications may be effective in increasing bladder capacity, decreasing bladder filling pressure, and improving bladder compliance. β3-adrenoceptor agonist may be considered in patients who are intolerant to anticholinergics. Intravesical Botox has been indirectly used to treat BPC in several studies examining the effect of Botox® on DO. In addition to increasing bladder capacity, Botox® has also been shown to improve bladder compliance [61].

In the setting of PPUI, when SUI surgery is considered, functional estimation bladder compliance becomes paramount. Any procedure that enhances bladder outlet such as male sling or AUS could increase bladder pressure that may be transmitted to the upper tracts, potentially placing kidneys at risk of chronic injury. Appropriate management of impaired compliance with the goal of reducing bladder pressures should be advocated prior to undertaking SUI surgery. Treatments should be delayed after multiple UDS evaluations to improve treatment success and to decrease the risk of undetermined upper urinary tract deterioration on the long run [62].

Data in literature about the safety of a male sling in terms of upper tract and renal function preservation in patients with PBC remain limited. Theoretically, a tight compressive sling may be contraindicated while a nonocclusive sling may represent a safer option. Several series showed that in this setting of patients, the trans-obturator device, PBC, is not predictive of worse continence outcome despite the incidence of renal failure or hydronephrosis during follow-up remains unspecified [63].

Whether PBC represents an absolute contraindication to AUS surgery in the PPUI, nonirradiated patient population remains an unanswered question. In general, worse continence outcomes should be expected in those with impaired bladder compliance on preoperative urodynamic studies despite several series failed to corroborate these findings [64].

Moreover, preservation of continence status after AUS surgery may also represents a sign of unestablished upper urinary tract damage. Despite no safe threshold detrusor pressures for AUS implantation have been recommended in patients with severely impaired bladder compliance, an AUS may still be considered. In these patients, periodic assessment of renal function as kidney ultrasound should be highly recommended. Additionally, these patients should be also advised to perform timed voiding to avoid maintenance of high bladder pressures [65].

Finally, in the sub-setting of patients with persistently elevated bladder pressures, who cannot perform timed voiding due to physical impairment, or who have evidence of preexisting renal deterioration, or who may not be suitable for SUI surgery, they should be advised on the protective role of PPUI as a "pop-off" mechanism, protecting indirectly their upper tracts [66].

In conclusion, stress urinary incontinence (SUI) remains the most common cause of PPUI, but bladder dysfunction in the form of DU, DO, and BPC represents combined causes of PPUI that must be carefully investigated. They may occur in the preoperative RP setting or they may arise de novo after surgery. Furthermore, they may appear alone or in combination with SUI. Irrespective of their nature, bladder dysfunctions may significantly affect the outcome of SUI surgery. Consequently, they should be treated on an individual basis. In summary, patients with SUI and DO are strongly recommended to have their DO treated first while patients with DU and SUI must be advised on their inability to void after sling positioning. Patients with BPC may need their compliance improved to prevent upper tract damage before considering SUI correction [67].

4.8 Bowel Dysfunction After RP

In the last decade, the transition to robotic radical prostatectomy (RARP) represented the main paradigm shift in the approach to the surgical management of prostate cancer (PCa) [1].

Although patients perceive that robotics will reduce perioperative complications, several series showed that RARP had a significantly higher frequency of genitourinary and miscellaneous medical complications during the first 90 days, while traditional open approach had a significantly higher risk of blood transfusions and prolonged hospitalization [68–70]. Regarding abdominal complications, several authors revealed a significantly higher risk of hernia and small bowel obstruction (SBO) among men treated by RARP. SBO represents a potentially major complication, which is often ensued by a lysis of adhesions (LOA). RARP is actually performed through a transperitoneal approach while the extraperitoneal route is limited to few centers worldwide [71].

Advantages in performing RARP via a transperitoneal approach include a wider working space and shorter time required to prepare the surgical field. However, disadvantages of this approach include unavoidable contact with bowels, which may directly or indirectly induce potential scarring or adhesions [72].

Only small series have investigated the risk of bowel complications after transperitoneal versus extraperitoneal RARP [73]. Extraperitoneal RARP is usually associated with significantly greater trocar insertion time but shorter console time, lower blood loss, shorter hospitalization, and shorter time for beginning an oral diet. However, irrespective of the surgical route considered, the rate of paralytic ileus in the RARP series appears negligible but logically increased in the transperitoneal series (extraperitoneal: 0–1% vs. transperitoneal: 4.5–6.7%) [74].

Concerning other types of bowel complications, RARP was also significantly associated with an increased risk of incision hernia. Several authors also suggested that transperitoneal RARP increases the amount of small bowel that would receive dosing of salvage radiation which might potentially impact the risk of subsequent abdominal complications in cases of recurrent prostate cancer [75–77].

Undoubtedly, intraperitoneal surgery leads to adhesions and represents the most common cause of small bowel obstruction (SBO), accounting for approximately half of all cases of SBO after gynecological, general, and urologic surgery [78]. Despite transperitoneal RARP may be associated with an increased risk of readmissions due to SBO and abdominal pain compared to extraperitoneal route, the risk of any abdominal complication at 5 years after surgery remains comparable suggesting that the risk of later events through the formation of adhesions and the frequency of these complications remains limited.

Furthermore, the best clinical "SBO definition" remains controversial. The most common exemplification is represented by "intolerance to solid diet," without specifying whether SBO was considered as mechanical or paralytic. Abdominal pain, nausea, and vomiting can be subclinical manifestations of SBO due to adhesions. According to current evidence, the cumulative incidence of readmission for SBO after RARP across series was negligible (0.4%) [79].

Potential causes leading to SBO have been hypothesized to be postoperative intra-abdominal adhesions. Possibly, additional factors related to the abdominal access may explain the increased risk of SBO and related readmissions. These include incarcerated trocar site hernia wound dehiscence and intra-abdominal urinary leakage [80]. These complications are related to bowel paralysis or incarceration. The exact frequency of trocar site hernia remains unknown. Finally, during the first year after RARP, there is a significantly increased risk of readmissions due to SBO and other intraperitoneal complications but not in the long term, as would be expected if RARP induced adhesions leading to SBO [81].

4.8.1 The Nightmare of Rectal Injury

Rectal injury (RI) remains a feared complication of RP with an incidence of 0.5–9%. It always represents a clinical dilemma for urologists. The opening of the bowel during prostatectomy converts the surgery from clean to contaminated. Therefore, the risk of septic complications increases, including wound infection, pelvic abscess, peritonitis, and recto-urinary fistula [82].

Current management strategies for bowel injury include extensive preoperative bowel preparation, perioperative and postoperative antibiotics, colostomy, and/or primary repair, with or without omental interposition between the rectum and vesicourethral anastomosis [83].

Most RI frequently occurs during the learning curve of RP, irrespective of the surgical approach considered. The risk factors include periprostatic fibrosis, previous prostate or rectal surgery, radiotherapy, previous hormonal therapy, and infection. The disease stage of locally advanced PCa tumors can also result in a difficult dissection and might result in RI during dissection of the undefined plane between the prostate and the rectum. Furthermore, extrafascial RP may also contribute to rectal injury due to the dissection plane being closer to the rectum and possible overconfidence while performing a standard nerve-sparing RP [84]. Prostate weight does not seem to have an impact on the incidence of RI. Other potential factors increasing the risk of rectourethral fistula have been reported, such as previous androgen deprivation therapy, pelvic fracture, and rectal surgery [85]. In patients with extensive bowel adhesions due to inflammatory disease, previous colorectal or pelvic surgeries including colostomy reversal might have an increased risk of rectal injury during RP while obesity seems to be a protective factor against rectal injuries. In this setting of patients, it is reasonable to assume that the perirectal adipose tissue may act as a physical barrier granting an additional protective space between the rectum and the prostate [86].

Common rectal injuries during minimally invasive RP usually occur during transection of the rectourethralis muscle and development of the rectal-prostatic plane. They are usually located near to the apex and the rectourethralis muscle. Notably, the incidence reported by using a trans-Douglas approach remains negligible (0.2%) [87]. To prevent this serious complication, dissection of the prostatic apex should be made carefully and sharply with cold scissors by dividing the rectourethral muscle from the posterolateral angle while the assistant keeps the rectum posteriorly with the tip of a suction device. Furthermore, adequate incision of the posterior layer of Denonvilliers' fascia is required to avoid entry into the perirectal fat after completing dissection of both seminal vesicles.

In cases of bowel injury unrevealed intraoperatively, thermal tissue damage from the different sealant device or of the monopolar current or inadvertent damage while changing instruments may play a role [88]. Sometimes, the rectal defect may have been temporarily sealed off by the thermal device, making it practically undetectable [89]. Bowel injury following minimally invasive surgery may have an unusual presentation and devastating sequelae, especially if unrecognized intraoperatively. Ileocolonic injuries may present postoperatively as primarily ileus and abdominal distention in the absence of peritoneal signs. Failure to recognize and promptly treat a bowel injury may result in higher rates of mortality and morbidity. If atypical acute abdomen develops postoperatively, prompt computerized tomography as immediate surgical exploration represents critical actions [82].

Most authors concur that antibiotic therapy and starvation may help the healing of a rectal injury in early postoperative care. However, it remains debatable whether managing rectal injury during prostatectomy requires a transitory/definitive bowel and/or urinary diversion, rectal repair, and interposition of healthy fat flap between the rectal repair and vesicourethral anastomosis [90].

In the past, a diverting colostomy was recommended while today, however, primary repair without a diverting colostomy is advocated in most cases. According to current clinical practice, the overall percentage of colostomy applied in cases with rectal injury ranged between 18% and 32%. A diverting colostomy is strongly recommended for cases of previous radiotherapy, inadequate repair, a tense suture line, poor tissue quality, a history of radiation to the pelvis, or significant fecal contamination in the field [91].

Preoperative preparation may be helpful in reducing bowel injuries, including preoperative group education, operative complication explanation, adequate bowel preparation, and antibiotics. Video recordings of each case may be also useful to identify problems in patients with bowel injury missed intraoperatively. Despite uncommon during RARP, RI can lead to severe postoperative complications. It can be managed robotically if early identified by a two-layer rectal wall closure. The best treatment remains injury prevention. Unrecognized bowel injury may have atypical presentation. Dissemination of the presentation and management of bowel injury as modifications to avoid complications might help to improve RARP outcomes [92].

Unfortunately, no preoperative measures focused to avoid the risk of RI or minimize its potential infective consequences could be currently recommended. In detail, no specific antibiotic prophylaxis is indicated for patients potentially at risk for RI. Mechanical bowel preparation does not positively affect perioperative morbidity associated with RI during RP and, therefore, it is usually omitted [93].

The management and prognosis of RI significantly differ by timing of detection. Intraoperative detection of RI has strongly been associated with a significantly decreased risk of severe postoperative complications and subsequent formation of an RUF. Consequently, all measures aimed at identifying the presence of RI intraoperatively should strongly be considered and applied in a standardized manner [94].

Careful dissection and development of the posterior plane between the prostate and rectal wall favoring the use of cold scissors and avoiding monopolar cautery close to the rectal wall, visualization of the periprostatic fat tissue during extrafascial posterior dissection, and minimal traction on the rectum wall in the presence of periprostatic adhesions might represent important tricks to reduce RI risk [95].

A probe or a sponge stick can be eventually placed in the rectum at the beginning of the surgical procedure to help the surgeon identify any rectal mucosal perforation. If RI is suspected, or in the presence of a visible thin rectal wall, the pneumatic test must always be done. After prostate removal, the pelvis should be irrigated to remove blood clots and to identify any actively bleeding vessels and then filled with standard saline solution. Air can be also insufflated into the rectum using the rectal probe. The detection of air bubbles escaping from the rectum is clearly due to the presence of a small rectal lesion. In absence of a preliminarily placed rectal probe, air can be insufflated into the rectum through a rectal Foley catheter while the pelvis is filled with irrigation fluid. Performing an intra-abdominal washing with a wide-spectrum antimicrobial irrigation may represent an option to minimize the risk of severe sepsis [82].

If RI occurs at the beginning of the procedure during the seminal vesicle dissection or at the development of the posterior plane between the prostate and the rectum wall, the lesion may be repaired at this stage before proceeding with further mobilization of the prostate. Regardless of the approach used, the rectal defect must be closed before completing the vesicourethral anastomosis. Usually, the rectal defect can be closed using absorbable (Monocryl or Vicryl) 2-0 or 3-0 sutures in two layers (mucosa and seromuscular). Interposition of viable and vascularized tissues such as omentum between the injured rectal wall and the vesicourethral anastomosis should strongly be considered to create a barrier improving the rectal wound healing [96].

Wherever omentum mobilization may result challenging (short omentum, previous surgery, or steep Trendelenburg position), a full-layer peritoneal graft obtained from the pelvic side wall can be used alternatively as a third layer to cover the area of RI. Colostomy should not be considered as the standard of care in all patients with intraoperatively detected RI. However, it should strongly be considered in patients with large rectal defects (>2 cm) and/or previous pelvic radiotherapy and/or previous BPH-related surgery and/or suspected PCa infiltration of the rectum [97]. A suction drain should be placed especially if the vesicourethral anastomosis is not watertight and if the suture line for RI repair remains under tension.

In the postoperative management, broad-spectrum antibiotic therapy is strongly recommended. Moreover, a longer catheterization time should strongly be considered (>2 weeks) and the catheter removal should be planned only after a negative cystogram. Nevertheless, 10% of patients with intraoperatively detected RI develop an RUF during the postoperative period. A consistent proportion of patients treated conservatively or surgically for RI develops an RUF in the following weeks.

In these cases, fecaluria, pneumaturia, and drainage of urine per anus pose a strong suspicion for the presence of an RUF. Usually, fecaluria is considered a poor prognostic sign. Retrograde urethrocystography, flexible or rigid urethrocystoscopy, and rectoscopy or colonoscopy should strongly be considered to plan the most appropriate surgical treatment. Although several approaches, including transperineal, transanal, transabdominal, transvesical, trans-sphincterial, or combined, have been proposed, there is no standardized treatment for RUF due to its low incidence [98, 99].

Nevertheless, the York-Mason technique is still considered the most appropriate according to its high success rate and low morbidity. Although several studies reported high success rates after the most popular surgical techniques, a recurrent RUF occurs and represents a very challenging issue in clinical practice because repeated surgical failures significantly increase morbidity and mortality in these patients [100–102].

Additionally, a recurrent RUF represents the greatest challenge for surgeons. Patients with a recurrent RUF who had previously undergone pelvic radiation therapy and/or those with unfavorable anatomical conditions (low bladder capacity) and/or a high risk of infective/general complications should be considered for permanent urinary and/or fecal diversion [103].

The potential occurrence of RI should always be discussed during the preoperative patient counseling and promptly investigated during surgery, especially when certain clinical factors are present, such as age >60 years and previous radiation therapy to the pelvis. Intraoperative detection and repair of RI during RP represent the most critical step to significantly decrease the risk of severe postoperative complications and subsequent RUF formation. Intraoperatively undetected RI can be responsible for severe infectious complications and can lead to an RUF in a high percentage of cases.

4.9 Sexual Dysfunction After RP

Erectile dysfunction (ED) represents a complex condition, dependent on central and peripheral mechanisms that involve spinal tracts, nerve bundles, vascular compartments, and smooth muscle cells. Spinal pathways involve both parasympathetic and sympathetic communication to promote and maintain a successful erection for sexual intercourse. The pelvic plexus located in the posterolateral wall of the prostate has been shown to provide autonomic innervation to the corpora cavernosa [104]. During RP, these cavernous nerves may be transected or damaged. Nerve-sparing techniques have provided a significant improvement in potency induction after RP. Nonetheless, ED is still evident in many patients even when undergoing bilateral Ns RP, suggesting that ED is not only attributable to a simple nerve injury. Several studies showed that patients undergoing bilateral Ns RP may have either arterial or venous insufficiency, suggesting an additional vascular nature of the pathophysiology of ED [105]. Indeed, maintenance of the appropriate oxygen levels in the corporal environment has been suggested to play a role in the prevention of corporal fibrosis. TGF-beta has been shown to promote corporal fibrosis in hypoxic states through the induction of collagen deposition in cavernosal smooth muscle cells. Vascular changes associated with RP may theoretically induce a hypoxic microenvironment which may result in cavernosal fibrosis [106]. Furthermore, the physiological neuropraxia after surgery may cause long-term low oxygen tension state in the penis, possibly resulting in smooth muscle apoptosis and fibrosis. These irreversible changes may induce a veno-occlusive status. Since these events are related to an initial nerve injury, the changes are most pronounced when a bilateral nerve damage is present. Therefore, the first step in preserving EF relies on the surgical technique chosen during RP. Regardless of the heterogeneity in potency definition, the sexual dysfunction at 12 and 24 months after RP ranges from 10% to 46% and 6% to 37%, respectively [107].

With the increasing proportion of young men undergoing RP, the importance of postoperative erectile recovery is gradually emerging [108]. Despite postoperative ED may recover gradually within 2 years or longer after RP, most patients are unlikely to return to their baseline erectile function [109]. This condition led to significant decrements in quality of life, self-cognition, and couple cohesion. In this context, penile rehabilitation was initially proposed to facilitate the recovery of erectile dysfunction after RP [110].

The main goal of penile rehabilitation is to restore satisfactory EF based on the enhancement of corpora cavernosa oxygenation and interruption of cavernous nerve injury-induced structural changes of the penile tissue [111]. Conventional recovery treatments offered for ED includes pelvic floor muscle training (PFMT), use of phosphodiesterase type 5 inhibitors (PDE5is), intracavernous injection of vasoactive substance (IC), vacuum erection devices, and a combination of these treatments [112]. More recently, psychotherapy intervention, stem cell therapy, low-intensity extracorporeal shockwave therapy (LiESWT), tacrolimus, and hyperbaric oxygenation therapy emerged as alternative therapies [113]. To date, major limitations and contrasting results from previous series hampered the elaboration of a guideline for clinical practice. Finally, surgical approach to implant a penile prosthesis is recommended as second-line therapy to patients that have failed medical therapy nor are satisfied with results and medications delivery routes [114].

First step of penile rehabilitation is to discuss exhaustively the occurrence of post-RP ED with every patient. Furthermore, it is paramount to assess EF using available questionnaires, such as International Index of Erectile Function (IIEF) and

Expanded Prostate Cancer Index Composite (EPIC), prior to and after the procedure to monitor EF recovery after RP [115]. Patients should be aware that post-RP ED can be permanent or temporary. They should be also informed of the relevant predictors of EF recovery, such as younger age, preoperative EF, bilateral Ns RP, and all penile rehabilitation methods. It is essential that patients figure out that timeframe recovery of postoperative EF can take many years. Finally, additional sexual changes should be clarified by the urologist, such as reduced libido, changes in orgasm, anejaculation, climacturia, and reduction of penile size [116].

Partner support seems to be positively associated with patient adherence to medical treatments for ED. Although the main goal of RP is oncological, for many patients, restoration of EF remains equally important. Psychological factors, such as relationship quality, depression, or anxiety, may play an important role for the postoperative couple's sexuality [117].

An historical study by Mulhall, dividing men who started penile rehabilitation early after RP (<6 months) from those who had delayed (>6 months) start in penile rehabilitation, showed significant improvement in EF domain score for the early group. Starting penile rehabilitation within 6 months of RP may offer benefits in improving overall EF but must be carried out in an individualized manner to assure safety and adherence to therapy [118]. More recently, several author studies have advocated a more precocious start of penile rehabilitation, starting PDE5-I use as soon as the catheter is removed [119].

Common adverse effects reported for PDE5-I include headache, flushing, nasal congestion, nasopharyngitis, and dyspepsia. Rare but serious reports of priapism have been seldom reported [120]. Despite nerve-sparing surgical techniques, PDE5-I are usually not very effective early after surgery, with 12–17% of responders after 6 months, because the cavernous nerves are injured intraoperatively and can take until 2 years to heal [121]. Unfortunately, ED post RP may not be completely attributed to acute nerve injury but rather to its chronic sequalae. The use of a strict definition for ED recovery remains, however, a urological dilemma [122].

4.9.1 Vacuum Erection Device (VED)

VED provides negative pressure to the penis, creating a passive engorgement of the corpora cavernosa. Men are advised to use a constrictor ring placed at the base of the penis to retain blood within the corpora in the early postoperative setting after RP [123]. Several series showed that 80% of patients that began early use of VED could have sexual intercourse, with a 55% sexual satisfaction rate [124]. After 9 months, 17% of men had spontaneous erections sufficient for vaginal intercourse, compared to 10% of men in the control group. Furthermore, a recent study demonstrated that PDE5-I or the combination of PDE5-I and VED were the only modalities able to increase EF recovery after surgery. Conversely, VED as single therapy failed to show improvement in postoperative EF recovery [125].

Evidence on VED efficacy was limited by a small sample size studies and by the heterogeneity in preoperative characteristics, where a significant proportion of the subjects already had ED before surgery [124]. An additional benefit that may result with daily use of a VED instead of PDE-5I is the preservation of penile length after RP as some studies suggest that no penile rehabilitation therapy may result in up to a 2 cm penile length reduction [126]. The most common side effects of VED are mild and include numbness, pain, and penile bruising. The use of the correct negative pressure should avoid most of these side effects. Men may also complain of lack of spontaneity and the sensation of a "cold" penis, in analogy to urethral surgery. Other rare complications such as leg spasms, testicular migration, and urethral bleeding have been occasionally reported [124].

4.9.2 Intracavernous Injection (IC)

IC therapy represents an important therapeutic option for men with ED. After administrated, the IC stimulate relaxation of the corpora cavernosa smooth muscle to induce an erection. The most common administered drugs are phentolamine, prostaglandin E1 (PGE1), and papaverine [127].

Phentolamine is an alpha-adrenergic antagonist that causes a decrease in peripheral vascular resistance and vasodilatation. On the other hand, PGE1 is an endogenous prostaglandin that decreases the influx of calcium within the penile vascular smooth muscle, leading to relaxation of trabecular smooth muscle, arterial dilation, blood entrapment, and erection. Papaverine is a direct-acting smooth muscle relaxant, causing the nonselective inhibition of PDE enzyme and direct inhibition of calcium channels. Among the benefits of IC, it does not involve irreversible procedures or the use of devices and has reproducible erection responses with tolerable side effects. Despite many advantages, some studies report a 11–31% drop-out rate, especially due to pain (11%) and lack of efficacy (9.7%) [128, 129].

Penile rehabilitation with IC was initially proposed by Montorsi et al. in 1997 [130]. Patients were initially given IC of alprostadil three times per week for 6 months and compared to patients without injections. 67% of men that received ICI reported spontaneous erections sufficient for intercourse, while 20% of men in the control group had spontaneous erections.

IC should be used between 4 and 10 min before intercourse and its effects will last for approximately 2 h after the injection. Before starting the treatment, men should be counseled about possible side effects and complications of IC. The most feared side effect is having prolonged and painful erections, also known as priapism. Other possible side effects include corporal fibrosis (2%, papaverine), hypotension and tachycardia (phentolamine), and prolonged penile pain [127].

4.9.3 Intraurethral Therapy with Suppository (MUSE)

Medicated urethral system for erections (MUSE) involves the formulation of alprostadil (PGE1) into a small intraurethral suppository that can be inserted into the urethra. Currently, the only available randomized study investigating MUSE for penile rehabilitation compared MUSE with daily sildenafil in a small series of patients showing no difference in EF 1 year after RP [131]. However, the lack of a placebo and a no-treatment group for comparison precludes proper analysis and comparison with other methods of penile rehabilitation in most of the studies published. Furthermore, flaws in the design with improper randomization preclude an unbiased analysis [132]. Finally, the median drop-out rate in the MUSE group due to lack of efficacy, reduced sexual interest, and adverse effects in all published series is attested around 32%. The most common adverse events reported of MUSE are local pain (29–41%), dizziness possibly associated to hypotension (1.9–14%), penile fibrosis, priapism (<1%), urethral bleeding (5%), and urinary tract infections (0.2%) [133].

4.10 Low-Intensity Extracorporeal Shockwave Therapy (Li-ESWT)

The principles of low-intensity ESWT (Li-ESWT) for erectile dysfunction (ED) were introduced by the pioneering clinical research work of Vardi et al. [134]. Li-ESWT results in an improvement of the intra-cavernosal pressure/mean arterial pressure ratio indicating an immediate improvement of erectile function. The positive effects of Li-ESWT on erectile function are potentiated by the concomitant use of PDE5i [135].

Li-ESWT can be successfully used for regenerative therapy even after tissue and functional damages have occurred after cavernous nerve injury in patients after RP [136]. Moreover, Li-ESWT might be an appropriate method to prevent or at least delay structural changes in the aging penis, finally resulting in deterioration of erectile function or penile shrinking [137].

The positive effects of Li-ESWT on cavernosal tissue and function in the preclinical setting as described earlier occurred with a great variation of total number of shockwaves, varying between 0.01 and 0.11 mJ/mm^2, shockwaves per session between 300 and 2000, and the total number of shockwaves between 300 and 24,000 depending on the investigational series considered and the shockwave machine used [138].

The huge heterogeneity in the treatment protocols and energies applied makes the interpretation and comparison of the results of all available studies difficult and leaves many questions open/unanswered regarding the best sources of energies, the optimum number of shockwaves per session, the optimum intervals between the sessions, and the optimum total number of shockwaves. Some studies in which different EFDs and different protocols were compared provided at least some evidence that a higher total number of shockwaves may result in a better outcome [139].

Nearly all published studies in ED have shown beneficial effects of Li-ESWT on a variety of parameters related to cavernosal/erectile function such as restoration of aging or damaged arteries/nerves and fibrotic tissue changes in the aging penis, including the impact of increased sympathetic activity in the aging man [140]. Furthermore, without any exception, in none of the published trials, relevant side effects of ESWT were observed so far [141].

Meanwhile, there is growing evidence in the literature that early initiation of rehabilitation strategies starting even with the time of RP may finally result in higher rates of preservation of functional cavernous tissue and therefore of potency [142]. Simultaneously with or immediately after RRP, administration of the PDE5i sildenafil, tadalafil, or vardenafil has proven to avoid most of the detrimental effects of cavernous neurotomy with the prevention of loss of smooth muscle cell and corporal fibrosis due to increase of collagen content [143].

Finally, there is granular evidence that the combination of ESWT with daily dosing PDE5i is clearly superior to ESWT alone. Nevertheless, regardless of indication, Li-ESWT on the penis should always be combined with daily dosing of a PDE5i, which standard dosage remains yet to be determined [144].

4.10.1 Penile Implant

Penile prosthesis represents the most effective therapeutic modality for severe refractory ED and provides reliable, on-demand, artificial erections with high satisfaction rates [145]. The two most common indications for the surgery remain organic ED (23.7%) and post-RP ED (21.2%). Although a high number of penile prostheses were implanted after RP for ED, only a small amount of post-RP patients would proceed with an early penile implant. The mean time from RP to prosthesis implantation reported was approximately 2.6 years [146]. Since the recovery from neuropraxia after RP with a nerve-sparing intent is usually time dependent, penile prosthesis implantation for post-RP ED is generally delayed for at least 1 year following the procedure, justifying the long timeframe between RP and the penile prosthesis implant. A recent study which evaluated predictors of penile prosthesis implant found that men after RP were of a younger age, African/American/Hispanic race, and unmarried [147].

The two currently available types of penile prostheses include malleable and inflatable devices (2 pieces or 3 pieces). The malleable device requires a less invasive procedure (since they have no reservoir) and results in a rigid penis, which may be manually concealed by bending the penis when desired. The 2-piece inflatable prosthesis can be an interesting option among patients who are at high-risk of complications with reservoir placement besides being easier to manipulate [148]. The 3-piece inflatable devices are usually preferred due to the more "natural" erections obtained and excellent rigidity besides mimicking the flaccid state of the penis but requiring higher manual dexterity. Attention should be given to the reservoir placement when performing the 3-piece inflatable prosthesis implant in patients with history of RP. The reservoir is usually placed in the space of Retzius, but if it remains obliterated due to previous pelvic surgery, the reservoir may be placed in the submuscular space, anterior to the transversalis fascia, using a separated incision or through the inguinal ring. A retroperitoneal placement of the reservoir may represent an option for specific cases when the abdominal wall condition precludes the conventional sites [149].

Satisfaction after a penile prosthesis implant is as high as 80% even when considering all functional aspects of the device, such as inflation, deflation, and rigidity. Further studies reported satisfaction rates with malleable prostheses higher than 90% and slightly higher when considering inflatable devices [150]. Despite the need for psychological and sexual adaptation after the penile prosthesis implant, patients experience a marked improvement in EF. In addition to an increase in the regularity of sexual activity and sexual satisfaction, there is also an improvement of mood and anxiety. The most important factors contributing to high level of satisfaction are rapid generation of erection, consistently optimal rigidity, negligible rate of postoperative complications, ease of concealment, cosmetic outcome, device function, ease of use, and of utmost importance, partner acceptance [151].

The two most important complications of penile prostheses surgery are represented by mechanical failure and infection [152]. Several improvements of the 3-piece prosthesis over time resulted in a mechanical failure rate of <5% after 5 years of follow-up [153]. Moreover, surgical techniques that decrease contact with the patient's skin associated with proper antibiotic prophylaxis reduced infection rates to 2–3% with primary implantation in low-risk patients and high-volume centers [154, 155]. Additionally, this therapy requires the ability to grasp and visualize the penis for appropriate use; therefore, either the patient or the partner needs to have a certain degree of hand dexterity for this therapeutic option to be effective. For men lacking such manual dexterity, a malleable penile device can be offered due to its simpler operability [156, 157].

References

1. Costello AJ. Considering the role of radical prostatectomy in 21st century prostate cancer care. Nat Rev Urol. 2020;17(3):177–88.
2. Haney CM, Kowalewski KF, Westhoff N, Holze S, Checcuci E, Neuberger M, et al. Robot-assisted versus conventional laparoscopic radical prostatectomy: a systematic review and meta-analysis of randomised controlled trials. Eur Urol Focus. 2023;9(6):930–7.
3. Donovan JL, Hamdy FC, Lane JA, Mason M, Metcalfe C, Walsh E, et al. Patient-reported outcomes after monitoring, surgery, or radiotherapy for prostate cancer. N Engl J Med. 2016;375(15):1425–37.
4. Lardas M, Liew M, van den Bergh RC, De Santis M, Bellmunt J, Van den Broeck T, et al. Quality of life outcomes after primary treatment for clinically localised prostate cancer: a systematic review. Eur Urol. 2017;72(6):869–85.
5. Holze S, Lemaire E, Mende M, Neuhaus P, Arthanareeswaran VKA, Truss MC, et al. Quality of life after robotic-assisted and laparoscopic radical prostatectomy: results of a multicenter randomized controlled trial (LAP-01). Prostate. 2022;82(8):894–903.
6. Walz J, Epstein JI, Ganzer R, Graefen M, Guazzoni G, Kaouk J, et al. A critical analysis of the current knowledge of surgical anatomy of the prostate related to optimisation of cancer control and preservation of continence and erection in candidates for radical prostatectomy: an update. Eur Urol. 2016;70(2):301–11. https://pubmed.ncbi.nlm.nih.gov/26850969/. [cited 2022 Feb 16].
7. Kadono Y, Nohara T, Kawaguchi S, Iwamoto H, Yaegashi H, Shigehara K, et al. Impact of pelvic anatomical changes caused by radical prostatectomy. Cancers (Basel). 2022;14(13):3050.

8. Hodges PW, Stafford RE, Hall L, Neumann P, Morrison S, Frawley H, et al. Reconsideration of pelvic floor muscle training to prevent and treat incontinence after radical prostatectomy. Urol Oncol Semin Orig Investig. 2020;38(5):354–71.
9. Asimakopoulos AD, Annino F, Colalillo G, Gaston R, Piechaud T, Mauriello A, et al. "Urethral-sparing" robotic radical prostatectomy: critical appraisal of the safety of the technique based on the histologic characteristics of the prostatic urethra. Curr Oncol. 2023;30(1):1065–76.
10. Wagaskar VG, Mittal A, Sobotka S, Ratnani P, Lantz A, Falagario UG, et al. Hood technique for robotic radical prostatectomy—preserving periurethral anatomical structures in the space of Retzius and sparing the pouch of Douglas, enabling early return of continence without compromising surgical margin rates. Eur Urol. 2021;80(2):213–21.
11. Kojima Y, Takahashi N, Haga N, Nomiya M, Yanagida T, Ishibashi K, et al. Urinary incontinence after robot-assisted radical prostatectomy: pathophysiology and intraoperative techniques to improve surgical outcome. Int J Urol. 2013;20(11):1052–63.
12. Geng E, Yin S, Yang Y, Ke C, Fang K, Liu J, et al. The effect of perioperative pelvic floor muscle exercise on urinary incontinence after radical prostatectomy: a meta-analysis. Int Braz J Urol. 2023;49(4):441–51.
13. Mungovan SF, Carlsson SV, Gass GC, Graham PL, Sandhu JS, Akin O, et al. Preoperative exercise interventions to optimize continence outcomes following radical prostatectomy. Nat Rev Urol. 2021;18(5):259–81.
14. Hennessey DB, Hoag N, Gani J. Impact of bladder dysfunction in the management of post radical prostatectomy stress urinary incontinence—a review. Trans Androl Urol. 2017;6(Suppl 2):S103–11. http://www.ncbi.nlm.nih.gov/pubmed/28791229. [cited 2024 Mar 12].
15. Peyronnet B, Brucker BM. Management of overactive bladder symptoms after radical prostatectomy. Curr Urol Rep. 2018;19(12):95.
16. Del Giudice F, Huang J, Li S, Sorensen S, Enemchukwu E, Maggi M, et al. Contemporary trends in the surgical management of urinary incontinence after radical prostatectomy in the United States. Prostate Cancer Prostatic Dis. 2023;26(2):367–73.
17. Rosier PFWM, Schaefer W, Lose G, Goldman HB, Guralnick M, Eustice S, et al. International continence society good urodynamic practices and terms 2016: urodynamics, uroflowmetry, cystometry, and pressure-flow study. Neurourol Urodyn. 2017;36(5):1243–60.
18. Porena M, Mearini E, Mearini L, Vianello A, Giannantoni A. Voiding dysfunction after radical retropubic prostatectomy: more than external urethral sphincter deficiency. Eur Urol. 2007;52(1):38–45.
19. Yao HH, Hoe V, Crump RT, Sengupta S, O'Connell HE, Carlson KV, et al. Impact of radical prostatectomy on bladder function as demonstrated on urodynamics study—a systematic review. Neurourol Urodyn. 2021;40(2):582–603.
20. Kadono Y, Ueno S, Yaegashi H, Ofude M, Izumi K, Maeda Y, et al. Urodynamic evaluation before and immediately after robot-assisted radical prostatectomy. Urology. 2014;84(1):106–11.
21. Gacci M, De Nunzio C, Sakalis V, Rieken M, Cornu J-N, Gravas S. Latest evidence on post-prostatectomy urinary incontinence. J Clin Med. 2023;12(3):1190. http://www.ncbi.nlm.nih.gov/pubmed/36769855. [cited 2024 Mar 12].
22. Pastore AL, Palleschi G, Illiano E, Zucchi A, Carbone A, Costantini E. The role of detrusor overactivity in urinary incontinence after radical prostatectomy: a systematic review. Minerva Urol e Nefrol. 2017;69(3):234–41.
23. Rahnama'i MS, Marcelissen T, Geavlete B, Tutolo M, Hüsch T. Current management of post-radical prostatectomy urinary incontinence. Front Surg. 2021;8:647656. http://www.ncbi.nlm.nih.gov/pubmed/33898508. [cited 2024 Mar 12].
24. Kim M, Park M, Shim M, Choi SK, Lee SM, Lee ES, et al. Effect of preoperative urodynamic detrusor overactivity on post-prostatectomy incontinence: a systematic review and meta-analysis. Int Urol Nephrol. 2016;48(1):53–63.

25. Thiruchelvam N, Cruz F, Kirby M, Tubaro A, Chapple CR, Sievert KD. A review of detrusor overactivity and the overactive bladder after radical prostate cancer treatment. BJU Int. 2015;116(6):853–61.
26. Lee DS, Lee S-J. Urodynamic evaluation of patients with localized prostate cancer before and 4 months after robotic radical prostatectomy. Sci Rep. 2021;11(1):3632.
27. Sakalis V, Gkotsi A. Do drugs work for OAB following prostate cancer surgery. Curr Drug Targets. 2020;21(15):1515–26.
28. Ervandian M, Djurhuus JC, Høyer M, Graugaard-Jensen C, Borre M. Long-term urodynamic findings following radical prostatectomy and salvage radiotherapy. Scand J Urol. 2018;52(1):20–6.
29. Song C, Lee J, Hong JH, Choo MS, Kim CS, Ahn H. Urodynamic interpretation of changing bladder function and voiding pattern after radical prostatectomy: a long-term follow-up. BJU Int. 2010;106(5):681–6.
30. Giannantoni A, Mearini E, Zucchi A, Costantini E, Mearini L, Bini V, et al. Bladder and urethral sphincter function after radical retropubic prostatectomy: a prospective long-term study. Eur Urol. 2008;54(3):657–64.
31. Zhou Z, Wang X, Li X, Liao L. Detrusor relaxing agents for neurogenic detrusor overactivity: a systematic review, meta-analysis and network meta-analysis. BJU Int. 2024;133(1):25–33.
32. Ficazzola MA, Nitti VW. The etiology of post-radical prostatectomy incontinence and correlation of symptoms with urodynamic findings. J Urol. 1998;160(4):1317–20.
33. Palmer C, Farhan B, Nguyen N, Zhang L, Do R, Nguyen DV, et al. Are electronic and paper questionnaires equivalent to assess patients with overactive bladder? J Urol. 2018,200(2):369–74.
34. Walter M, Leitner L, Betschart C, Engeler DS, Freund P, Kessler TM, et al. Considering non-bladder aetiologies of overactive bladder: a functional neuroimaging study. BJU Int. 2021;128(5):586–97.
35. Dmochowski RR, Newman DK, Rovner ES, Zillioux J, Malik RD, Ackerman AL. Patient and clinician challenges with anticholinergic step therapy in the treatment of overactive bladder: a narrative review. Adv Ther. 2023;40(11):4741–57.
36. Bapir R, Bhatti KH, Eliwa A, Garcia-Perdomo HA, Gherabi N, Hennessey D, et al. Efficacy of overactive neurogenic bladder treatment: a systematic review of randomized controlled trials. Arch Ital Urol Androl. 2022;94(4):492–506.
37. Ribeiro L, Leung LY, Tan N, Low ZY, Nagarajah M, Ahmed G, et al. Predictors for adverse events following intravesical botulinum toxin injections in men. Neurourol Urodyn. 2023;42(7):1499–505.
38. Habashy D, Losco G, Tse V, Collins R, Chan L. Botulinum toxin (OnabotulinumtoxinA) in the male non-neurogenic overactive bladder: clinical and quality of life outcomes. BJU Int. 2015;116:61–5.
39. Shabataev V, Saadat SH, Elterman DS. Management of erectile dysfunction and LUTS/incontinence: the two most common, long-term side effects of prostate cancer treatment. Can J Urol. 2020;27(27):17–24.
40. Quek ML, Barry P, Stein JP, Lieskovsky G, Ginsberg DA. Combined radical prostatectomy and bladder augmentation for concomitant prostate cancer and detrusor instability. Urology. 2005;65(5):964–7.
41. Colaco M, Osman NI, Karakeçi A, Artibani W, Andersson KE, Badlani GH. Current concepts of the acontractile bladder. BJU Int. 2018;122(2):195–202.
42. Gajewski JB, Drake MJ. Neurological lower urinary tract dysfunction essential terminology. Neurourol Urodyn. 2018;37:S25–31.
43. Oszczudlowski M, Cymbalista G, Bilski K, Dobruch J. Detrusor underactivity after radical prostatectomy: a prospective observational study. Neurourol Urodyn. 2024;43(3):638–45. http://www.ncbi.nlm.nih.gov/pubmed/38273775. [cited 2024 Mar 12].
44. Ahmed A, Farhan B, Vernez S, Ghoniem GM. The challenges in the diagnosis of detrusor underactivity in clinical practice: a mini-review. Arab J Urol. 2016;14(3):223–7. http://www.ncbi.nlm.nih.gov/pubmed/27547465. [cited 2024 Mar 12].

45. Osman NI, Chapple CR, Abrams P, Dmochowski R, Haab F, Nitti V, et al. Detrusor underactivity and the underactive bladder: a new clinical entity? A review of current terminology, definitions, epidemiology, aetiology, and diagnosis. Eur Urol. 2014;65(2):389–98.
46. Osman NI, Esperto F, Chapple CR. Detrusor underactivity and the underactive bladder: a systematic review of preclinical and clinical studies. Eur Urol. 2018;74(5):633–43.
47. Wang J, Ren L, Liu X, Liu J, Ling Q. Underactive bladder and detrusor underactivity: new advances and prospectives. Int J Mol Sci. 2023;24(21):15517.
48. Chung DE, Dillon B, Kurta J, Maschino A, Cronin A, Sandhu JS. Detrusor underactivity is prevalent after radical prostatectomy: a urodynamic study including risk factors. Can Urol Assoc J. 2013;7(1–2):E33–7. http://www.ncbi.nlm.nih.gov/pubmed/22277630. [cited 2024 Mar 12].
49. Jura YH, Comiter CV. Urodynamics for postprostatectomy incontinence: when are they helpful and how do we use them? Urol Clin North Am. 2014;41(3):419–27.
50. Krughoff K, Peterson AC. Clinical and urodynamic determinants of earlier time to failure for the artificial urinary sphincter. Urology. 2023;176:200–5.
51. Comiter CV, Dobberfuhl AD. The artificial urinary sphincter and male sling for postprostatectomy incontinence: which patient should get which procedure? Investig Clin Urol. 2016;57(1):3–13.
52. Rizvi IG, Ravindra P, Pipe M, Sohawon R, King T, Belal M. The AdVance™ male sling: does it stand the test of time? Scand J Urol. 2021;55(2):155–60.
53. Welk BK, Herschorn S. The male sling for post-prostatectomy urinary incontinence: a review of contemporary sling designs and outcomes. BJU Int. 2012;109(3):328–44.
54. Koch GE, Kaufman MR. Male stress urinary incontinence. Urol Clin North Am. 2022;49(3):403–18.
55. Lee UJ, Ward JB, Feinstein L, Matlaga BR, Martinez-Miller E, Bavendam T, et al. National trends in neuromodulation for urinary incontinence among insured adult women and men, 2004–2013: the Urologic Diseases in America Project. Urology. 2021;150:86–91.
56. Johnson TM, Vaughan CP. Urological function and dysfunction in aging: diagnosis and treatment. Handb Clin Neurol. 2019;167:495–509.
57. Cho SY, Yi JS, Oh SJ. The clinical significance of poor bladder compliance. Neurourol Urodyn. 2009;28(8):1010–4.
58. Gomha MA, Boone TB. Voiding patterns in patients with post-prostatectomy incontinence: urodynamic and demographic analysis. J Urol. 2003;169(5):1766–9.
59. Abrar M, Pindoria N, Malde S, Chancellor M, DeRidder D, Sahai A. Predictors of poor response and adverse events following botulinum toxin A for refractory idiopathic overactive bladder: a systematic review. Eur Urol Focus. 2021;7(6):1448–67.
60. Zeng X, Shen SH, Shen H, Luo DY. Statistical process control for the analysis of quality control in urodynamics: a potential new approach for quality review of urodynamics. Neurourol Urodyn. 2023;42(1):289–96.
61. Oszczudłowski M, Bilski K, Kozikowski M, Dobruch J. De novo detrusor underactivity and other urodynamic findings after radical prostatectomy: a systematic review. Medicina. 2022;58(3):381.
62. Crivellaro S, Morlacco A, Bodo G, Agro' EF, Gozzi C, Pistolesi D, et al. Systematic review of surgical treatment of post radical prostatectomy stress urinary incontinence. Neurourol Urodyn. 2016;35(8):875–81.
63. Toia B, Leung LY, Saigal R, Solomon E, Malde S, Taylor C, et al. Is pre-operative urodynamic bladder function the true predictor of outcome of male sling for post prostatectomy incontinence? World J Urol. 2021;39(4):1227–32.
64. Smith WJ, VanDyke ME, Venishetty N, Langford BT, Franzen BP, Morey AF. Surgical management of male stress incontinence: techniques, indications, and pearls for success. Res Rep Urol. 2023;15:217–32. http://www.ncbi.nlm.nih.gov/pubmed/37366389. [cited 2024 Mar 12].

65. Bole R, Hebert KJ, Gottlich HC, Bearrick E, Kohler TS, Viers BR. Narrative review of male urethral sling for post-prostatectomy stress incontinence: sling type, patient selection, and clinical applications. Transl Androl Urol. 2021;10(6):2682–94.
66. Barski D, Gerullis H, Otto T. Review of surgical implant procedures for male incontinence after radical prostatectomy according to IDEAL framework. Updates Surg. 2017;69(3):327–38.
67. Hennessey DB, Hoag N, Gani J. Impact of bladder dysfunction in the management of post radical prostatectomy stress urinary incontinence—a review. Transl Androl Urol. 2017;6(Suppl 2):S103–11. https://pubmed.ncbi.nlm.nih.gov/28791229/. [cited 2024 Mar 3].
68. Terry RS, Gupta M, Su LM. Complications of robot-assisted radical prostatectomy. In: Robot genitourin surgery. 2nd ed; 2018. p. 493–505.
69. Basiri A, de la Rosette JJ, Tabatabaei S, Woo HH, Laguna MP, Shemshaki H. Comparison of retropubic, laparoscopic and robotic radical prostatectomy: who is the winner? World J Urol. 2018;36(4):609–21.
70. Cheng E, Gereta S, Zhang TR, Zhu A, Basourakos SP, McKernan C, et al. Same-day discharge vs inpatient robotic-assisted radical prostatectomy: complications, time-driven activity-based costing, and patient satisfaction. J Urol. 2023;210(6):856–64.
71. Loeb S, Meyer CP, Krasnova A, Curnyn C, Reznor G, Kibel AS, et al. Risk of small bowel obstruction after robot-assisted vs open radical prostatectomy. J Endourol. 2016;30(12):1291–5.
72. Stolzenburg JU, Rabenalt R, Do M, Lee B, Truss MC, McNeill A, et al. Complications of endoscopic extraperitoneal radical prostatectomy (EERPE): prevention and management. World J Urol. 2006;24(6):668–75.
73. Goldberg IP, Chang SL, Kundu SD, Chung BI, Singer EA. Impact of inflammatory bowel disease on radical prostatectomy outcomes and costs of care. Prostate Int. 2021;9(2):66–71. http://www.ncbi.nlm.nih.gov/pubmed/34386447. [cited 2024 Mar 12].
74. Ozdemir AT, Altinova S, Koyuncu H, Serefoglu EC, Cimen IH, Balbay DM. The incidence of postoperative ileus in patients who underwent robotic assisted radical prostatectomy. Cent Eur J Urol. 2014;67(1):19–24.
75. Hampson A, Raj N, Lingamanaicker V, Thakur S, Shan GM, Prasad V, et al. Serum cytokine levels as markers of paralytic ileus following robotic radical prostatectomy at different pneumoperitoneum pressures. Curr Urol. 2021;15(2):91–4. http://www.ncbi.nlm.nih.gov/pubmed/34168526. [cited 2024 Mar 12].
76. Petersen PM, Cook AD, Sydes MR, Clarke N, Cross W, Kynaston H, et al. Salvage radiation therapy after radical prostatectomy: analysis of toxicity by dose-fractionation in the RADICALS-RT trial. Int J Radiat Oncol Biol Phys. 2023;117(3):624–9.
77. Huelster HL, Laviana AA, Joyce DD, Huang LC, Zhao Z, Koyama T, et al. Radiotherapy after radical prostatectomy: effect of timing of postprostatectomy radiation on functional outcomes. Urol Oncol Semin Orig Investig. 2020;38(12):930.e23–32.
78. Lundström KJ, Folkvaljon Y, Loeb S, Axelson AB, Stattin P, Nordin P. Small bowel obstruction and abdominal pain after robotic versus open radical prostatectomy. Scand J Urol. 2016;50(3):155–9.
79. Ávila M, Patel L, López S, Cortés-Sanabria L, Garin O, Pont À, et al. Patient-reported outcomes after treatment for clinically localized prostate cancer: a systematic review and meta-analysis. Cancer Treat Rev. 2018;66:23–44.
80. Adejoro O, Gupta P, Ziegelmann M, Weight C, Konety B. Effect of minimally invasive radical prostatectomy in older men. Urol Oncol Semin Orig Investig. 2016;34(5):234.e1–11.
81. Soto-Palou FG, Sánchez-Ortiz RF. Outcomes of minimally invasive inguinal hernia repair at the time of robotic radical prostatectomy. Curr Urol Rep. 2017;18(6):43.
82. Romito I, Giannarini G, Rossanese M, Mucciardi G, Simonato A, Ficarra V. Incidence of rectal injury after radical prostatectomy: a systematic review and meta-analysis. Eur Urol open Sci. 2023;52:85–99. http://www.ncbi.nlm.nih.gov/pubmed/37213241. [cited 2024 Mar 12].
83. Canda AE, Tilki D, Mottrie A. Rectal injury during radical prostatectomy: focus on robotic surgery. Eur Urol Oncol. 2018;1(6):507–9.

84. Mandel P, Linnemannstöns A, Chun F, Schlomm T, Pompe R, Budäus L, et al. Incidence, risk factors, management, and complications of rectal injuries during radical prostatectomy. Eur Urol Focus. 2018;4(4):554–7.
85. Luciani LG, Mattevi D, Puglisi M, Processali T, Anceschi U, Lauro E, et al. Robotic-assisted radical prostatectomy following colo-rectal surgery: a user's guide. J Robot Surg. 2022;16(1):189–92.
86. Luciani LG, Mattevi D, Mantovani W, Cai T, Chiodini S, Vattovani V, et al. Retropubic, laparoscopic, and robot-assisted radical prostatectomy: a comparative analysis of the surgical outcomes in a single regional center. Curr Urol. 2017;11(1):36–41. http://www.ncbi.nlm.nih.gov/pubmed/29463975. [cited 2024 Mar 12].
87. Luchaichana N, Ramart P. Management of rectal injury and rectourinary fistula from radical prostatectomy. Urol Ann. 2023;15(1):31–4. http://www.ncbi.nlm.nih.gov/pubmed/37006220. [cited 2024 Mar 12].
88. Awwad JT, Isaacson K. The harmonic scalpel: an intraoperative complication. Obstet Gynecol. 1996;88(4 II Suppl):718–20.
89. Liang J, Xing H, Chang Y. Thermal damage width and hemostatic effect of bipolar electrocoagulation, LigaSure, and Ultracision techniques on goat mesenteric vessels and optimal power for bipolar electrocoagulation. BMC Surg. 2019;19(1):147.
90. Barashi NS, Pearce SM, Cohen AJ, Pariser JJ, Packiam VT, Eggener SE. Incidence, risk factors, and outcomes for rectal injury during radical prostatectomy: a population-based study. Eur Urol Oncol. 2018;1(6):501–6.
91. Masuda T, Kinoshita H, Nishida S, Kawa G, Kawakita M, Matsuda T. Rectal injury during laparoscopic radical prostatectomy: detection and management: skills and pitfalls. Int J Urol. 2010;17(5):492–5.
92. Wedmid A, Mendoza P, Sharma S, Hastings RL, Monahan KP, Walicki M, et al. Rectal injury during robot-assisted radical prostatectomy: incidence and management. J Urol. 2011;186(5):1928–33.
93. Kheterpal E, Bhandari A, Siddiqui S, Pokala N, Peabody J, Menon M. Management of rectal injury during robotic radical prostatectomy. Urology. 2011;77(4):976–9.
94. Roberts WB, Tseng K, Walsh PC, Han M. Critical appraisal of management of rectal injury during radical prostatectomy. Urology. 2010;76(5):1088–91.
95. Harpster LE, Rommel FM, Sieber PR, Breslin JA, Agusta VE, Huffnagle HW, et al. Incidence and management of rectal injury associated with radical prostatectomy in a community based urology practice. J Urol. 1995;154(4):1435–8.
96. Watts A, Kocher NJ, Pauli E, Raman JD. Endoscopic closure of a large rectovesical fistula following robotic prostatectomy. J Endourol Case Rep. 2020;6(3):139–42. http://www.ncbi.nlm.nih.gov/pubmed/33102710. [cited 2024 Mar 12].
97. Kanehira E, Tanida T, Kanehira AK, Takahashi K, Obana Y, Iwasaki M, et al. A new technique to repair vesicorectal fistula: overlapping rectal muscle plasty by transanal endoscopic surgery. Urol Int. 2021;105(3–4):309–15.
98. Massalou D, Chetrus-Mariage D, Baqué P. York-Mason repair of recto-urethral fistula. J Visc Surg. 2015;152(3):185–8.
99. Rogers P, Delgado Z, Garoufalia Z, Horesh N, Gefen R, Wexner SD. Gracilis muscle interposition for recurrent recto-urethral fistula: how we do it—a video vignette. Color Dis. 2023;25(12):2462–3.
100. Cathelineau X, Sanchez-Salas R, Flamand V, Barret E, Galiano M, Rozet F, et al. Surgery illustrated surgical atlas: the York Mason operation. BJU Int. 2010;106(3):436–47.
101. Falavolti C, Sergi F, Shehu E, Buscarini M. York Mason procedure to repair iatrogenic rectourinary fistula: our experience. World J Surg. 2013;37(12):2950–5.
102. Joshi HMN, Vimalachandran D, Heath RM, Rooney PS. Management of iatrogenic recto-urethral fistula by transanal rectal flap advancement. Color Dis. 2011;13(8):918–20.
103. Moretto G, Casaril A, Inama M. Use of biological mesh in trans-anal treatment for recurrent recto-urethral fistula. Int Urol Nephrol. 2017;49(9):1605–9.

104. Feng D, Tang C, Liu S, Yang Y, Han P, Wei W. Current management strategy of treating patients with erectile dysfunction after radical prostatectomy: a systematic review and meta-analysis. Int J Impot Res. 2022;34(1):18–36.
105. Lima TFN, Bitran J, Frech FS, Ramasamy R. Prevalence of post-prostatectomy erectile dysfunction and a review of the recommended therapeutic modalities. Int J Impot Res. 2021;33(4):401–9.
106. Goh HJ, Sung JM, Lee KH, Jo JK, Kim KN. Efficacy of phosphodiesterase type 5 inhibitors in patients with erectile dysfunction after nerve-sparing radical prostatectomy: a systematic review and meta-analysis. Transl Androl Urol. 2022;11(2):124–38. http://www.ncbi.nlm.nih.gov/pubmed/35280664. [cited 2024 Mar 12].
107. Marchioni M, de Francesco P, Castellucci R, Papalia R, Sarikaya S, Gomez Rivas J, et al. Management of erectile dysfunction following robot-assisted radical prostatectomy: a systematic review. Minerva Urol Nefrol. 2020;72(5):543–54.
108. Asker H, Yilmaz-Oral D, Oztekin CV, Gur S. An update on the current status and future prospects of erectile dysfunction following radical prostatectomy. Prostate. 2022;82(12):1135–61.
109. Hansen ST, Lund M, Ostergaard LD, Lund L. Role of regenerative therapies on erectile dysfunction after radical prostatectomy. Int J Impot Res. 2021;33(4):488–96.
110. Moretti TBC, Reis LO. The paradox of erectile dysfunction data after radical prostatectomy. Int Braz J Urol. 2022;48(5):880–2.
111. Gandaglia G, Suardi N, Cucchiara V, Bianchi M, Shariat SF, Roupret M, et al. Penile rehabilitation after radical prostatectomy: does it work? Transl Androl Urol. 2015;4(2):110–23. http://www.ncbi.nlm.nih.gov/pubmed/26816818. [cited 2024 Mar 12].
112. Liu C, Lopez DS, Chen M, Wang R. Penile rehabilitation therapy following radical prostatectomy: a meta-analysis. J Sex Med. 2017;14(12):1496–503.
113. Clavell-Hernández J, Wang R. The controversy surrounding penile rehabilitation after radical prostatectomy. Transl Androl Urol. 2017;6(1):2–11. http://www.ncbi.nlm.nih.gov/pubmed/28217445. [cited 2024 Mar 12].
114. Kohn TP, Rajanahally S, Hellstrom WJG, Hsieh TC, Raheem OA. Global trends in prevalence, treatments, and costs of penile prosthesis for erectile dysfunction in men. Eur Urol Focus. 2022;8(3):803–13.
115. Bock M, Burns RT, Pereira TA, Bernie HL. A contemporary review of the treatments and challenges associated with penile rehabilitation after radical prostatectomy including a proposed optimal approach. Int J Impot Res. 2023;36(5):480–5. https://pubmed.ncbi.nlm.nih.gov/37853240/. [cited 2024 Mar 12].
116. Kannady C, Clavell-Hernandez J. Orgasm-associated urinary incontinence (climacturia) following radical prostatectomy: a review of pathophysiology and current treatment options. Asian J Androl. 2020;22(6):549–54.
117. Nicolai M, Urkmez A, Sarikaya S, Fode M, Falcone M, Albersen M, et al. Penile rehabilitation and treatment options for erectile dysfunction following radical prostatectomy and radiotherapy: a systematic review. Front Surg. 2021;8:636974. https://pubmed.ncbi.nlm.nih.gov/33738297/. [cited 2024 Mar 12].
118. Hatzimouratidis K, Burnett AL, Hatzichristou D, McCullough AR, Montorsi F, Mulhall JP. Phosphodiesterase type 5 inhibitors in postprostatectomy erectile dysfunction: a critical analysis of the basic science rationale and clinical application. Eur Urol. 2009;55(2):334–47.
119. Baccaglini W, Pazeto CL, Corrêa Barros EA, Timóteo F, Monteiro L, Saad Rached RY, et al. The role of the low-intensity extracorporeal shockwave therapy on penile rehabilitation after radical prostatectomy: a randomized clinical trial. J Sex Med. 2020;17(4):688–94. https://pubmed.ncbi.nlm.nih.gov/32007430/. [cited 2024 Mar 12].
120. Capogrosso P, Salonia A, Briganti A, Montorsi F. Postprostatectomy erectile dysfunction: a review. World J Mens Health. 2016;34(2):73–88. http://www.ncbi.nlm.nih.gov/pubmed/27574591. [cited 2024 Mar 13].
121. McMahon CG. Current diagnosis and management of erectile dysfunction. Med J Aust. 2019;210(10):469–76.

122. Salonia A, Bettocchi C, Boeri L, Capogrosso P, Carvalho J, Cilesiz NC, et al. European Association of Urology guidelines on sexual and reproductive health—2021 update: male sexual dysfunction [Formula presented]. Eur Urol. 2021;80(3):333–57.
123. Wang C-M, Wu B-R, Xiang P, Xiao J, Hu X-C. Management of male erectile dysfunction: from the past to the future. Front Endocrinol (Lausanne). 2023;14:1148834. http://www.ncbi.nlm.nih.gov/pubmed/36923224. [cited 2024 Mar 13].
124. Pirola GM, Naselli A, Maggi M, Gubbiotti M, Rubilotta E, Jeremy Yuen-Chun T, et al. Vacuum erection device for erectile function rehabilitation after radical prostatectomy: which is the correct schedule? Results from a systematic, scoping review. Int J Impot Res. 2023;36(3):194–200. http://www.ncbi.nlm.nih.gov/pubmed/37085734. [cited 2024 Mar 13].
125. Zhang M, Che JZ, Liu YD, Wang HX, Huang YP, Lv XG, et al. A prospective randomized controlled study on scheduled PDE5i and vacuum erectile devices in the treatment of erectile dysfunction after nerve sparing prostatectomy. Asian J Androl. 2022;24(5):473–7.
126. Sultana A, Grice P, Vukina J, Pearce I, Modgil V. Indications and characteristics of penile traction and vacuum erection devices. Nat Rev Urol. 2022;19(2):84–100.
127. Lea AP, Bryson HM, Balfour JA. Intracavernous alprostadil: a review of its pharmacodynamic and pharmacokinetic properties and therapeutic potential in erectile dysfunction. Drugs Aging. 1996;8(1):56–74.
128. Yiou R, Cunin P, De La Taille A, Salomon L, Binhas M, Lingombet O, et al. Sexual rehabilitation and penile pain associated with intracavernous alprostadil after radical prostatectomy. J Sex Med. 2011;8(2):575–82.
129. Gromicho A, Costa P, Araújo D, Pereira D, Ferraz L. Sexual rehabilitation with intracavernous alprostadil after radical prostatectomy: outcomes from a nursing program. Arch Ital Urol Androl. 2021;93(4):404–7.
130. Montorsi F, Guazzoni G, Strambi LF, Da Pozzo LF, Nava L, Barbieri L, et al. Recovery of spontaneous erectile function after nerve sparing radical retropubic prostatectomy with and without early intracavernous injections of alprostadil: results of a prospective, randomized trial. J Urol. 1997;158(4):1408–10.
131. Costa P, Potempa AJ. Intraurethral alprostadil for erectile dysfunction: a review of the literature. Drugs. 2012;72(17):2243–54.
132. Hanchanale V, Eardley I. Alprostadil for the treatment of impotence. Expert Opin Pharmacother. 2014;15(3):421–8.
133. Nik-Ahd F, Shindel AW. Pharmacotherapy for erectile dysfunction in 2021 and beyond. Urol Clin North Am. 2022;49(2):209–17.
134. Gruenwald I, Kitrey ND, Appel B, Vardi Y. Low-intensity extracorporeal shock wave therapy in vascular disease and erectile dysfunction: theory and outcomes. Sex Med Rev. 2013;1(2):83–90. http://www.ncbi.nlm.nih.gov/pubmed/27784587. [cited 2024 Mar 13].
135. Porst H. Review of the current status of low intensity extracorporeal shockwave therapy (Li-ESWT) in erectile dysfunction (ED), Peyronie's disease (PD), and sexual rehabilitation after radical prostatectomy with special focus on technical aspects of the different marketed ESWT devices including personal experiences in 350 patients. Sex Med Rev. 2021;9(1):93–122.
136. Raheem OA, Natale C, Dick B, Reddy AG, Yousif A, Khera M, et al. Novel treatments of erectile dysfunction: review of the current literature. Sex Med Rev. 2021;9(1):123–32.
137. Bocchino AC, Pezzoli M, Martínez-Salamanca JI, Russo GI, Lo Giudice A, Cocci A. Low-intensity extracorporeal shock wave therapy for erectile dysfunction: myths and realities. Investig Clin Urol. 2023;64(2):118–25.
138. Matthew AN, Rogers DE, Grob G, Blottner M, Kodama S, Krzastek SC. The use of low-intensity extracorporeal shockwave therapy in management of erectile dysfunction following prostate cancer treatment: a review of the current literature. Transl Androl Urol. 2023;12(6):1023–32. https://pubmed.ncbi.nlm.nih.gov/37426598/. [cited 2024 Mar 13].
139. Sighinolfi MC, Eissa A, Bellorofonte C, Mofferdin A, Eldeeb M, Assumma S, et al. Low-intensity extracorporeal shockwave therapy for the management of postprostatectomy erectile dysfunction: a systematic review of the literature. Eur Urol open Sci. 2022;43:45–53. https://pubmed.ncbi.nlm.nih.gov/35928730/. [cited 2024 Mar 13].

140. Ladegaard PBJ, Mortensen J, Skov-Jeppesen SM, Lund L. Erectile dysfunction a prospective randomized placebo-controlled study evaluating the effect of low-intensity extracorporeal shockwave therapy (LI-ESWT) in men with erectile dysfunction following radical prostatectomy. Sex Med. 2021;9(3):100338. https://pubmed.ncbi.nlm.nih.gov/33789173/. [cited 2024 Mar 13].
141. Hatzichristou D. Low-intensity extracorporeal shock waves therapy (LI-ESWT) for the treatment of erectile dysfunction: where do we stand? Eur Urol. 2017;71(2):234–6.
142. Pai R, Ory J, Delgado C, Ramasamy R. Energy-based therapies for erectile dysfunction: current and future directions. Urol Clin North Am. 2021;48(4):603–10. https://pubmed.ncbi.nlm.nih.gov/34602179/. [cited 2024 Mar 13].
143. Cocci A, Fassio G, Migliorini F, Cito G, Antonelli A, Verrienti P, et al. Low-intensity extracorporeal shock wave therapy (Li-ESWT) for priapism-induced erectile dysfunction in young patients: the first case series. Int J Impot Res. 2022;34(3):277–9. https://pubmed.ncbi.nlm.nih.gov/33820979/. [cited 2024 Mar 13].
144. Vardi Y, Appel B, Jacob G, Massarwi O, Gruenwald I. Can low-intensity extracorporeal shockwave therapy improve erectile function? A 6-month follow-up pilot study in patients with organic erectile dysfunction. Eur Urol. 2010;58(2):243–8.
145. Baird BA, Parikh K, Broderick G. Penile implant infection factors: a contemporary narrative review of literature. Transl Androl Urol. 2021;10(10):3873–84. http://www.ncbi.nlm.nih.gov/pubmed/34804829. [cited 2024 Mar 13].
146. Cocci A, Cito G, Romano A, Larganà G, Vignolini G, Minervini A, et al. Radical prostatectomy and simultaneous penile prosthesis implantation: a narrative review. Int J Impot Res. 2020;32(3):274–80.
147. Shah T, Wang R. A review of factors affecting patient satisfaction with inflatable penile prosthesis. Sex Med Rev. 2021;9(2):350–7.
148. Chung E. Penile prosthesis implant: scientific advances and technological innovations over the last four decades. Transl Androl Urol. 2017;6(1):37–45. http://www.ncbi.nlm.nih.gov/pubmed/28217449. [cited 2024 Mar 13].
149. La Croce G, Schifano N, Pescatori E, Caraceni E, Colombo F, Bettocchi C, et al. Which patient may benefit the most from penile prosthesis implantation? Andrology. 2022;10(8):1567–74.
150. Shen C, Jain K, Shah T, Schaefer E, Zhou S, Fried D, et al. Relationships between erectile dysfunction, prostate cancer treatment type and inflatable penile prosthesis implantation. Investig Clin Urol. 2022;63(3):316–24. https://pubmed.ncbi.nlm.nih.gov/35534219/. [cited 2024 Mar 13].
151. Scherzer ND, Dick B, Gabrielson AT, Alzweri LM, Hellstrom WJG. Penile prosthesis complications: planning, prevention, and decision making. Sex Med Rev. 2019;7(2):349–59.
152. Carvajal A, Henry GD. Prevention of penile prosthesis infection. Curr Urol Rep. 2022;23(5):75–81. https://pubmed.ncbi.nlm.nih.gov/35247139/. [cited 2024 Mar 13].
153. Smelser AM, Vandyke ME, Nealon SW, Badkhshan S, Langford BT, Peedikayil J, et al. Mechanical indications for inflatable penile prosthesis revision: analysis and implications for revision surgery. J Sex Med. 2023;20(7):1044–51.
154. Swanton A, Munarriz R, Gross M. Updates in penile prosthesis infections. Asian J Androl. 2020;22(1):28–33.
155. Pineda M, Burnett AL. Penile prosthesis infections—a review of risk factors, prevention, and treatment. Sex Med Rev. 2016;4(4):389–98.
156. Chung E, Wang J. State-of-art review of current malleable penile prosthesis devices in the commercial market. Ther Adv Urol. 2023;15:17562872231179008. http://www.ncbi.nlm.nih.gov/pubmed/37465318. [cited 2024 Mar 13].
157. Knoll P, Rai S, Talluri S, Bezinque A, Micciche R, Rao G, et al. A survey of usage of penile prosthesis. J Sex Med. 2020;17(11):2287–90.

Neurophysiological Testing After Prostatectomy and Urinary Diversion

5

Gianluca Sampogna, Sabrina Ravaglia, and Michele Spinelli

Key Points

- Neurophysiological testing (i.e., sacral reflexes, pudendal nerve terminal motor latency, pudendal somatosensory evoked potential, perineal sympathetic skin response) may offer a series of methods to measure and assess the nervous system function after pelvic surgery, which are rarely considered.
- Neurophysiological tests may confirm findings on physical examination, establish the possible functional correlates of perineal dysfunction, and measure the severity of nervous system involvement.
- Neurophysiological tests may provide some prognostic clues as regards the likelihood of recovery and the type of therapeutic intervention each time indicated (i.e., pharmacological treatment, physical therapy, sacral neuromodulation, urethral sling, or artificial urinary sphincter).
- This research field is still in its infancy and future studies should fill the gaps highlighted in this chapter.

5.1 Introduction

Pelvic surgery (e.g., radical prostatectomy [RP], radical cystectomy [RC], urinary diversion [UD]) may be associated with urinary incontinence (UI) and sexual disturbances, like erectile dysfunction (ED), anorgasmia, and climacturia [1–3].

G. Sampogna (✉) · M. Spinelli
Neuro-Urology, Unipolar Spinal Unit, Niguarda Hospital, Milan, Italy
e-mail: gianluca.sampogna@unimi.it; michele.spinelli@ospedaleniguarda.it

S. Ravaglia
Stroke Unit, IRCCS Mondino Foundation, Pavia, Italy
e-mail: sabrina.ravaglia@mondino.it

G. Lamberti, C. De Nunzio (eds.), *Bladder, Bowel and Sexual Dysfunctions Rehabilitation after Radical Prostatectomy*, Urodynamics, Neurourology and Pelvic Floor Dysfunctions, https://doi.org/10.1007/978-3-031-76341-0_5

These adverse effects are usually assessed subjectively through questionnaires, like the International Consultation on Incontinence Questionnaire–Urinary Incontinence (ICIQ-UI) and the International Index of Erectile Function (IIEF) (see Chap. 11) [4, 5]. In contrast, neurophysiological testing (NT) may offer a series of methods to measure and assess the nervous system function after pelvic surgery, which are rarely considered [6].

The scope of this chapter is to present the basics of NT and report the evidence about its use after pelvic surgery. Considering the primordiality of this research field, the authors want to highlight the potentials and the gaps to fill with future studies in the future.

5.2 Neurophysiological Testing

NT may be divided into tests assessing (a) efferent motor innervation (i.e., pudendal nerve terminal motor latency [PTML], needle/surface perineal electromyography [EMG], motor evoked potentials); (b) somatosensory afferents (i.e., pudendal somatosensory evoked potentials [pSSEPs], penile sensory conduction velocity, perineal sensory threshold); (c) autonomic nervous system (i.e., perineal sympathetic skin response, assessing sympathetic fibers); and (d) spinal sacral reflexes, assessing both afferent sensory and efferent motor fibers, together with spinal cord interneurons [7]. Table 5.1 illustrates the main NT methods, which pathways are

Table 5.1 Summary of neurophysiological pelvic floor testing methods

Test	Method	Anatomical pathway	Outcome measures	Pros & cons
Needle EMG	Concentric needle examination of pelvic floor muscles (EAS, BC, EUS)	Somatic motor (sacral alpha-motor neurons)	Insertion activity Presence of spontaneous activity (denervation) Ability to activate muscle voluntarily, recruitment pattern MUAP: Waveform, amplitude, duration, phases Quantitative automated analysis of MUPs	Localization of a motor lesion Axonal vs. demyelinating damage Timing of damage Severity of damage (extent of denervation, recruitment pattern) Localization and assessment of EUS technically difficult in males

(continued)

Table 5.1 (continued)

Test	Method	Anatomical pathway	Outcome measures	Pros & cons
EMG surface polygraphy	Surface EMG activity (BC, auxiliary muscles)	Somatic motor (sacral alpha-motor neurons)	Amplitude/ frequency of pelvic floor myoelectric activity during rest and maximal contraction Use of auxiliary muscles/ efficiency to contract pelvic muscles isolated and sufficiently	Information about recruitment pattern only Requires needle EMG to exclude denervation
Sacral reflexes: BCR	Stimulation of dorsal penile nerve (anode distal) with pulses 0.1–0.2 ms, at pain intensity Registration by needle electrodes at the bulbocavernous muscles	Sacral reflex arc	Latency (28–42 ms) Amplitude (>10 μV) Persistence Interside difference in latency (<3 ms)	Assesses both the peripheral branches (sensory afferent and motor efferent) of the sacral reflex and the conus Localization of the lesion and of the type of fiber involved requires integration with other tests

(continued)

Table 5.1 (continued)

Test	Method	Anatomical pathway	Outcome measures	Pros & cons
Sacral reflexes: PUR, PAR	Stimulation as in BCR Registration at EUS and EAS	Sacral reflex arc	Latency (28–42 ms)	Assesses both the peripheral branches (sensory afferent and motor efferent) of the sacral reflex and the conus Localization of the lesion and of the type of fiber involved requires integration with other tests Continuous tonic activity of EAS/EUS obstacles detection of latency
Pudendal somatosensory evoked potential	Stimulation: Dorsal base of penis, bilaterally, with square wave pulses of 0.1 or 0.2 ms, 2–3 times over threshold Recording: Needle electrodes at Cz = −Fz Responses are amplified and averaged Three tracings are usually superimposed to determine the consistency of the response	Pudendal sensory fibers, central somatosensory pathway from sacral region to the cortex	Sensory threshold Latency Amplitude Consistency	Assessment of pudendal nerve sensory afferent fibers, sacral spinal cord, CNS lesions Localization of the lesion (central or peripheral) requires integration with other tests (i.e., BCR)
Pudendal motor evoked potentials	Magnetic stimulation of lumbosacral roots/ transcranial magnetic stimulation	Sacral roots, sacral plexus, and pudendal motor fibers, central motor pathway from the cortex to the sacral muscles	Latency	Sacral motor neurons Central motor conduction Unavailable in non-research centers

(continued)

Table 5.1 (continued)

Test	Method	Anatomical pathway	Outcome measures	Pros & cons
PTML	St. Mark's method	Pudendal nerve distal motor fibers	Latency of the CMAP Amplitude of CMAP	Low sensibility/specificity Only fastest motor fibers
Pudendal SSR	Stimulation: Median nerve, electric (or other types) Recording: Perineal skin, palm, foot	Postganglionic sympathetic efferent fibers, thoracolumbar sympathetic chain	Latency (side to side or perineal to feet comparison)	Integrity of sympathetic pathway Rapid habituation
Dorsal nerve of penis	Conduction velocity, with or without pharmacological erection	Peripheral sensory fibers	Conduction velocity	Technical errors of measurement
Pudendal nerve terminal sensory latency	Stimulation: Pudendal nerve within the rectum Recording: Sensory potential at the penis	Peripheral sensory fibers	Conduction velocity	

BCR bulbocavernous reflex, *CMAP* compound muscle action potential, *CNS* central nervous system, *EAS* external anal sphincter, *EMG* electromyography, *EUS* external urethral sphincter, *MUAP* motor unit action potential, *MUPs* motor unit potentials, *PAR* pudendal-anal reflex, *PTML* pudendal nerve terminal motor latency, *PUR* pudendal-urethral reflex, *SSR* sympathetic skin response

assessed by each test, and the meaning of any detected changes. We decide to describe only tests with definite or probable diagnostic or prognostic value, omitting those without established reliability [8]. Since many pathways overlap, the combination of different tests may help clarify whether there is a neurological damage, as well as the site of the lesion and the type of involved fibers, and the severity of nervous system damage.

5.2.1 Pudendal Nerve Terminal Motor Latency

PTML assesses the conduction of the fastest distal sacral motor nerve fibers within the pudendal nerve. The stimulation is performed with the St. Mark's technique, with the index finger close to the ischial spine of each side at 4 and 8 o'clock of the external anal sphincter (EAS) as depicted in Fig. 5.1 [9]. The compound muscle action potential (CMAP) is registered at the EAS (inferior hemorrhoidal branch) or at the bulbocavernous (BC) muscle (perineal branch). The outcome parameter is latency, while amplitude of the CMAP is considered less reliable. PTML may be

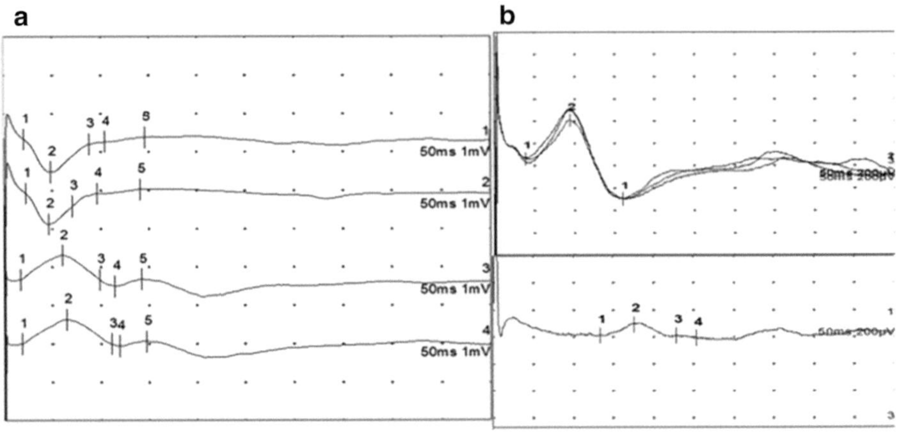

Fig. 5.1 (**a**) Pudendal nerve terminal motor latency (PTML), right side (upper traces) and left side (lower traces), normal values, as obtained with the St. Mark's pudendal electrode. (**b**) PTML normal latency and amplitude on the right side (upper trace) compared with increased latency and low amplitude on the left side

used to test for motor response in patients with suspected complete denervation of sacral/post-sacral segments, including the terminal perineal branches.

The St. Mark's electrode is a bipolar stimulating electrode fixed onto a gloved index finger, with the recording pair placed 8 cm proximally at the base of the index finger. Since the latency is very short (about 2 ms), it is unlikely that this represents the 8 cm conduction within the pudendal nerve, while it is more likely that the terminal pudendal nerve branches or pelvic floor muscles are stimulated directly, near their motor points. Bipolar perianal stimulation and recording of BC, EAS, and external urethral sphincter (EUS) muscles by concentric needle may be more reliable; using this technique, a latency of PTML of about 4.7–5.1 ms is obtained.

5.2.2 Electromyography

Concentric needle EMG may be used for qualitative or quantitative evaluation of motor unit potentials (MUPs) from pelvic floor muscles [10]. For addressing possible neurological damage post RP, the evaluation of the EUS or BC muscles, tested bilaterally, is especially useful. However, examination of male EUS is technically difficult, due to its small muscle bull, and since it requires a "blind" needle insertion in the perineum, with guidance by the investigator's finger in the rectum: Detection of continuous firing activity on relaxation indicates that the muscle has been correctly localized. In case of abnormal finding of both BC and EUS, recording of the EAS may be used to exclude (if normal) or confirm (if abnormal) a concomitant more proximal damage (sacral or post-sacral but proximal to the perineal nerve division).

Outcome measures of needle EMG include observation of insertion and spontaneous activity (signs of denervation); evaluation of tonic "basal" activity (for EUS/EAS); evaluation of activity during cough and during voluntary contraction; and observation of MUP parameters, including morphology, amplitude, duration, pattern of recruitment, and % of polyphasic potentials, globally representing reinnervation signs and giving information about the timing (acute, subacute, chronic) of the lesion. Evaluation of spontaneous activity in the EUS may be difficult due to the typical continuous firing of muscle activity in sphincters: In this situation, concomitant examination of the BC, that is silent on relaxation, is useful. Evaluation of activity pattern requires subjective collaboration to assess moderate intensity and maximal voluntary contraction, reflex contraction (e.g., by coughing), as well as the ability to contract perineal muscles independent of the co-activation of auxiliary (abdominal/thigh/gluteal) muscles.

The EMG signal is usually analyzed qualitatively, but quantitative techniques (i.e., multi-MUP analysis) are also available.

Surface EMG polygraphy consists in recording (usually for 10 s or more) EMG activity of the pelvic floor and of auxiliary muscles during rest and during maximal contraction [11]. This test provides information regarding maximal, minimal, and median amplitude and frequency of myoelectric activity during rest and during maximal contraction and efficiency to contract pelvic muscles isolated and sufficiently versus use of auxiliary muscles.

In summary, EMG evaluation of perineal muscles may help establish the anatomical site of muscle damage (depending on the involved muscles), the timing of neurological damage (depending on the presence of signs of denervation, concomitant denervation and reinnervation, or reinnervation only), and its severity (complete vs. partial denervation, recruitment pattern) and thus may be especially useful for prognostic purposes. To evaluate sphincter disturbances post RP and UD, the EUS would be the logical choice, but the BC, also providing information about the distal pudendal nerve/perineal branch, is usually analyzed for convenience since it is more easily accessible; moreover, unlike EUS, the BC may give information about the laterality of damage.

5.2.3 Pudendal Somatosensory Evoked Potentials

pSSEPs assess the integrity of the somatosensory pathway from the penis to the sensory cortex (Cz:Fz) [12]. Stimulation is performed by a bipolar handheld surface electrode (cathode proximal), placed on the proximal dorsal aspect of the penis, where the dorsal nerve of the penis (DNP), branch of the pudendal nerve, runs bilaterally, without fiber crossing in the midline. Thus, right and left trunks are stimulated separately. The sensitive threshold is the lowest perceptible current at the stimulation point and may also provide useful information about sensory damage. Indeed, although not an NT in the strict sense, electrical threshold provides useful information about perineal sensory function and is highly reproducible, if the patient collaborates. Stimulation with high frequency (>20 Hz) and duration of 0.5–1 ms is

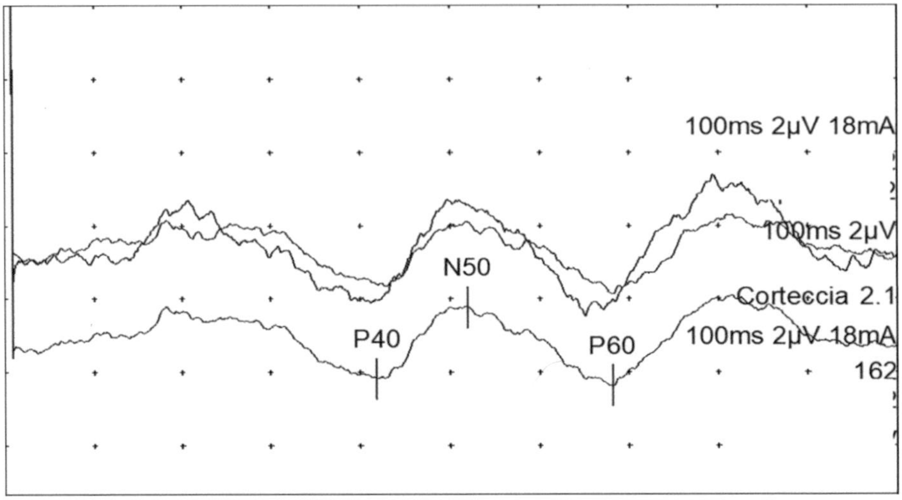

Fig. 5.2 Pudendal somatosensory evoked potentials. Cortical potentials to stimulation of the pudendal nerve, with the typical W shape. After the onset, the response follows a downward deflection (P40: first positive peak) and an upward deflection (N50: first negative peak). The second positive (P60) follows. The latency of the responses is usually measured at P40 response. The amplitude of the response is measured between the first peak-to-peak distance (P40-N50)

suggested, since more easily perceived. Stimulation intensity for SSEPs is set 2–4 times above threshold, depending on patient's tolerance. Latency of the first positive response (P1 or P40), amplitude, and reproducibility are assessed as outcomes (Fig. 5.2). Comparison with tibial SSEPs may help localize the site of damage in case of abnormal pudendal cortical response, as well as to exclude concomitant disorders. Comparison of pSSEPs response with sacral reflex may also help for localization purposes: If sacral reflexes are normal, altered pSSEPs usually indicate suprasacral lesions.

5.2.4 Sacral Reflexes

These tests measure the integrity of the reflex arc by stimulating a distal site and measuring the time it takes for the reflex contraction of the superficial perineal muscles [13]. After electrical stimulation of somatic sensory afferents, and after synapsing in the central nervous system by a polysynaptic pathway, efferent fibers carry the response to the skeletal muscle under study through the pudendal nerve. The most useful method to assess the anterior perineum is the *bulbocavernous reflex (BCR)*, in which the penile nerve is stimulated, and registration occurs at the BC. The *pudendal-anal reflex* and the *urethral-anal reflex* may be also assessed: the first with stimulation of penile nerve and registration at the EAS and the second by stimulating the perineal nerve at the EUS and registering at EAS. However, the BCR is preferred since, compared to EAS and EUS, the BC can be completely relaxed and thus the onset of the reflex is not obscured by continuous muscle fiber activity typical of sphincters.

The BCR explores the integrity of the pudendal nerve along its entire course through the peripheral and central nervous system (spinal interneurons, cord segment S2–4). The dorsal penile nerve is usually stimulated electrically (anode distal) with pulses 0.1–0.2 ms duration and at least three times above the sensory threshold. Needle or surface electrodes are placed at the BC muscle to register the reflex motor response. Elicitability of the response and its latency (R1, 28–42 ms, not influenced by patient height; with increase in stimulation intensity, an R2 response is also obtained) are the main outcome parameters (Fig. 5.3); interside difference in latency, amplitude, and persistence can be also assessed. For distal damage, as expected as deriving from pelvic surgery, significant (>3 ms) interside difference in latency may be more informative and sensitive to detect localized neurological damage compared to single unilateral latency values.

5.2.5 Perineal Sympathetic Skin Response

The only established NT to assess perineal autonomic (sympathetic) nerve fibers is the recording of the sympathetic skin response (SSR) [14]. SSR is a reflex consisting in myelinated sensory afferents, complex central integration (thoracolumbar trunk T10-L1), and a sympathetic efferent with postganglionic unmyelinated C-fibers. An electrical pulse (but also a noxious or other stimuli) with intensity three times above the sensory threshold is delivered, usually to the median nerve, and responses are recorded at the palm/feet and in the perineal area, by surface electrodes that register the variation in activity of skin sudomotor glands. After a latency

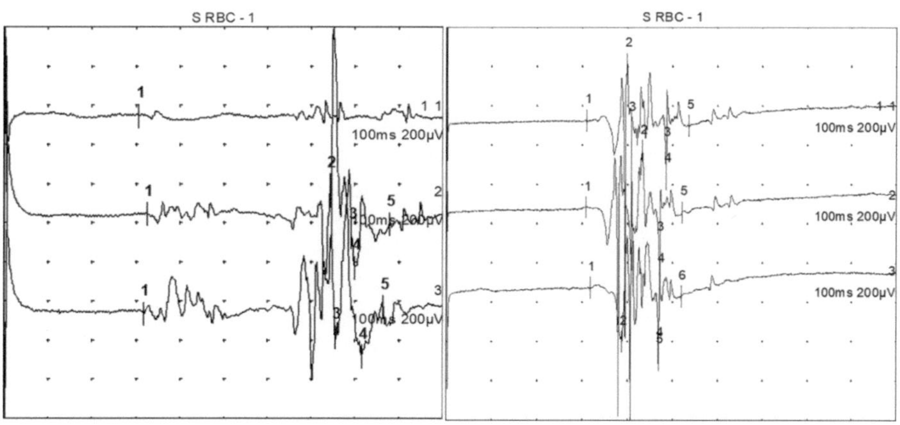

Fig. 5.3 Traces of a normal bulbocavernosus reflex (BCR). The first early oligosynaptic response, R1, occurs with a latency of 31–38 ms. With increase in stimulus intensity (right trace), a polysynaptic R2 response with increased latency and duration appears. The separation between the two components blurs at very strong stimulations

of 1.5–2.3 s, a perineal response, passing through the thoracolumbar sympathetic chain, is observed, and comparison with latencies obtained at the hand/foot and at the perineum may help localize the lesion distally to the thoracolumbar spinal segment, i.e., at a postganglionic level. The response rapidly habituates and has variable shape and amplitude so that only absent SSR is considered abnormal.

5.3 Evidence Acquisition

To collect and present studies concerning neurophysiological testing after RP and UD, the authors performed a literature search using PubMed, Cochrane Library, Scopus, and Web of Science databases in December 2022. The search was conducted by typing the following terms: *neurophysiological testing, neurophysiological test, neurophysiological investigation, electrophysiology, electromyography, sacral reflexes, pudendal nerve terminal motor latency, pudendal somatosensory evoked potential, perineal sympathetic skin response, sacral neuromodulation, prostatectomy, urinary diversion, and cystectomy*.

Two authors (GS and SR) independently screened the articles by title, abstract, and keywords and selected the ones to report based on the interest for the readers, study methodology, and novelty. Any disagreements were solved by discussion or with the opinion of the senior author (MS). Only full-text articles were considered. We decided not to include data from single case reports, replies to papers, and congress abstract proceedings as they usually lack the completeness of data required. Unpublished reports were not considered eligible. The search was limited to studies written in English and involving humans.

5.4 Evidence Synthesis

Our search highlighted few papers studying the analyzed topic. In particular, RP was deeply considered, while RC and UD were not included. The study quality was low. Table 5.2 illustrates the studies which utilized NT to assess perineal disturbances after pelvic surgery and summarizes the main findings [15–22].

The causes of perineal dysfunction after RP are not completely understood and may be multifactorial, including both "anatomical" changes (alteration of bladder neck, alteration of the bladder viscoelastic properties, shortening of the membranous urethra) and neurological causes (EUS muscle damage or damage of distal pudendal nerves). NT documentation of neurological damage after pelvic surgery, its severity, and its clinical correlates has been addressed by a few studies only.

One of the first published studies by Zermann et al. (2000) evaluated prospectively 18 patients before and after RP [23]. The outcomes of neuro-urological investigations (sacral reflexes, voluntary pelvic floor contraction and relaxation) and needle EMG showed no significant changes in the pre-/postoperative phases. Only by using surface EMG polygraphy, changes of activation patterns during pelvic floor contraction (decreased mean and medium frequency) could be found shortly

Table 5.2 Literature data on neurophysiological testing of the pelvic floor after radical prostatectomy

Author, year (study design)	Cases (age [years])	Type of NT	Clinical outcome assessed/ other testing	Result	Timing of testing
Catarin, 2008 (prospective)	46 (41–79, mean: 63)	SSEP, pudendo-anal and pudendo-urethral and urethra-anal reflex	Urinary incontinence/–	Postoperative increase in the urethro-anal reflex sensory threshold and latency possibly indicates autonomic dysfunction No variation in SSEP and any reflexes latencies	Pre surgery and 6 months after
Gerbaud, 2019 (prospective)	22 (mean: 66)	Simultaneous surface EMG of EAS and EIC during cough. Quantitative EMG of EAS	Urinary incontinence/–	Increased latency between the onset of EIC EMG and EAS EMG during cough	Not specified, however <1 year
Hacad, 2015 (prospective)	38 (63 ± 5.7)	Surface EMG	Urinary incontinence/–	No correlation between EMG abnormalities and urinary symptoms	6 months
Shefi, 2010 (retrospective)	20 (51–71, mean: 61)	BCR	Erectile dysfunction, response to sildenafil/–	Increase in latency predictive of sildenafil response; increase in latency and reduced amplitude predictive of no response; patients with normal BCR had no erectile dysfunction	3–6 months after surgery
Turmel, 2019 (prospective)	40	Pudendal terminal motor latency, EMG urethral sphincter, BCR, pudendal SSEP	Perineal pain, erectile dysfunction, urinary incontinence/–	Either abnormality without clear clinical correlation	Duration of the chronic pain: 2.7 ± 2.2 years
Ventimiglia, 2015 (retrospective)	79 (51–77, mean: 66)	Pudendal SSEP, perineal EMG	Urinary incontinence/ urodynamics	Increased SSEP latency and reduced amplitude; EMG incompetence in contraction or denervation, classifying outcome as neurapraxia/axonotmesis	4 and 24 months after surgery
Yildiz, 2021 (prospective)	26 (51–74, mean: 64)	Conduction velocity of dorsal penile nerve	Erectile dysfunction	Slowing of dorsal penile nerve sensory conduction	3–6 months after surgery
Zermann, 2000 (prospective)	18 (51–72, mean: 62)	Surface EMG polygraphy	Urinary incontinence/ urodynamics	Immediately after surgery: "Myoelectrical activity breaks" (short losses of amplitude during contraction); inefficiency to contract pelvic muscles isolated and sufficiently Normalization at 6 months	Before intervention, immediately after and 6 months later

BCR bulbocavernous reflex, *EAS* external anal sphincter, *EIC* external intercostal muscle, *EMG* electromyography, *SSEP* somatosensory evoked potential after surgery but not 6 months later. The authors speculated about a central disturbance of fine muscle function control: Neurophysiological events, caused by surgical dissection and an inflammatory reaction due to the healing process, would contribute to altered processing within the central nervous system (increased afferent inputs to the spinal cord dorsal horn), like a barrage of nociceptive information. According to the authors, the appreciation of these mechanisms, well studied in neuroscience and pain research, would offer a better understanding of surgery-related short- and long-term morbidity after pelvic surgery.

Electrodiagnostic evaluation of the BCR proved to be a valid predictor of response to sildenafil in ED after RP [18]. After at least 3 months after RP, patients with normal bulbocavernosus reflex latency (BCRL) and amplitude (BCRA) regained spontaneous erections, although insufficient for vaginal penetration, and presented a good response to 100 mg sildenafil. Patients with prolonged BCRL with normal BCRA did not present spontaneous erections and regained erections using sildenafil. Patients with prolonged BCRL and low BCRA lacked spontaneous erections and failed sildenafil trials, achieving erections using intracavernosal injections (ICI) of 10 μg prostaglandin E1 (PGE1).

Catarin et al. (2008) evaluated 44 patients within 6 months after surgery [15]. The pudendo-anal and pudendo-urethral reflexes were unchanged postoperatively (*P* value = 0.93 and 0.09, respectively), demonstrating that afferent and efferent pudendal innervation to this pelvic region was not affected by the surgery. Autonomic afferent denervation of the membranous urethral mucosa was found in 77.3% of patients, as demonstrated by a postoperative increase in the urethro-anal reflex sensory threshold and urethro-anal reflex latency (*P* value <0.001 and 0.0007, respectively). One patient required 3 pads daily and 23 showed urinary leakage, even if just 5 cases needed 1 pad per day. Afferent autonomic denervation at the membranous urethral mucosa was found in 91.7% of patients with urinary leakage. Among 10 cases with preserved urethro-anal reflex latency, 80% of patients were continent.

Yiou et al. (2012) assessed the value of the measurement of penile thermal and vibratory sensory thresholds to reflect cavernous nerve damage caused by RP [23]. Penile sensory thresholds for warm (*P* value <0.0001) and cold (*P* value <0.0001) sensations significantly increased after non-nerve-sparing RP but not after nerve-sparing RP. Vibration threshold only increased after transperineal non-nerve-sparing RP (*P* value = 0.031). Erectile Dysfunction Symptom Score (EDSS) values were significantly increased in all groups of patients 2 months after surgery.

Ventimiglia et al. analyzed retrospectively 79 patients with UI, 4 and 24 months after RP, by pudendal SSEPs and perineal EMG, disclosing increased SSEPs latency and reduced amplitude, as well as EMG incompetence in contraction and denervation [20]. Grouping of patients according to NT results allowed the authors to predict the best treatment option (anticholinergics, physical treatment, biofeedback, trans-obturator tape sling or artificial urinary sphincter for nonresponders due to severe neurological damage).

Yildiz et al. detected slowing of nerve conduction velocity of the dorsal penile nerve in 26 patients suffering from ED 3–6 months after RP [21].

Turmel et al. analyzed 40 patients with various perineal disturbances (pain, ED, UI) after RP by extensive NT including PTML, EMG of EUS, BCR, and pudendal SSEPs; the authors could not detect any clear correlation between NT abnormalities and type of clinical dysfunction [19].

In summary, the few studies addressing this issue differ as regards the target symptom addressed (urinary disturbances, ED, perineal pain) and how it was scored, the timing of NT after surgery, and the tests each time utilized. The aim of the studies also differs: some authors pointing at the speculation about the mechanisms of neurological damage and the type of fibers involved while others focusing on prognostic clues. A systematic assessment of NT after RP, its clinical counterpart (if any), correlation with preoperative data (type of surgery, prostate volume), comparison with clinical scores, and other functional investigations (i.e., urodynamics), as well as the mechanisms and severity of the neurological damage, the correct timing of NT, and its usefulness for prognostic purposes, is lacking till now.

In the event of post-RP perineal disturbances, the anatomical site of the possible neurological damage is already known and expected to involve the terminal portion of the pudendal nerve; the etiology is also known and may be furtherly clarified with imaging. Thus, NT should focus on excluding concomitant superimposed damage at more proximal levels (possibly highlighted by a distal damage), as well as to assess the severity of damage and the type of fiber mainly involved. Thus, NT may be helpful to confirm a clinical suspect of postsurgical neurological damage, establish its severity (complete vs. partial; axonal vs. demyelinating/compressive), and assess the type of nerve fibers mainly involved (motor vs. somatosensory vs. autonomic). This information may reveal relevant for predicting prognosis and possible treatment strategies (pharmacological, physical treatment, neurostimulation/neuromodulation) although current indications in this sense are lacking.

Guidelines as regards the best NT to predict long-term prognosis or a positive response to neuromodulation are also currently lacking. Only a few studies focused on the correlation between sacral dysfunction and NT results while there are no literature data about the utility of NT as predictors of response to neuromodulation.

We propose to consider the systematic assessment of a combination of the more reliable NTs (EMG of BC, BCR, pSSEPs, sensory threshold), focusing on relevant parameters, correlation with clinical scores, and correlation with long-term prognosis. Together with these tests that provide information about the functional status of the peripheral nervous system, morphological techniques (i.e., magnetic resonance imaging [MRI], computed tomography [CT], ultrasound imaging) may be useful to exclude concomitant anatomical causes. MRI, in particular Diffusion Tensor Imaging technique (DTI), may offer optimal representation of the widely distributed periprostatic plexus so that, if validated, it may help guide nerve-sparing RP [24].

5.5 Sacral Neuromodulation

Sacral neuromodulation (SNM) is a treatment for sacral area dysfunctions. In particular, approved indications are represented by overactive bladder, chronic nonobstructive urinary retention, and fecal incontinence [25]. SNM consists of the placement of a quadripolar electrode along the nerve roots passing through the S3 foramen to modulate the electrical activity of nerves controlling bladder, bowel, and genito-sexual functions. This electrode is connected to an implantable pulse generator (IPG), located in a subcutaneous buttock pocket. Since this therapy is expensive and not appropriate for all patients, most patients undergo a Peripheral Nerve Evaluation (PNE) test, based on the placement of a monopolar temporary electrode for a few days to 2 weeks [26]. This electrode comes out of the skin and is linked to an external nerve stimulator (ENS). If there is a ≥ 50% symptom improvement with PNE, the patient is addressed to the implant of the definitive system.

Stress UI (SUI) is not an approved indication for SNM. However, the placement of the aforementioned electrode along the pudendal nerve may stimulate the efferent component of this nerve improving symptoms [27]. By our tertiary referral center for SNM, the Niguarda Hospital, Milan, Italy, the chronic stimulation of pudendal nerve was tested in five patients suffering from SUI for at least 12 months after RP from January 2000 to December 2022. PNE test resulted in a significant symptom improvement in 2 out of 5 (40%) of cases. Responders were addressed to the implant of the definitive system. The other patients were addressed to different SUI treatments like urethral sling ($n = 1$) and artificial urinary sphincter ($n = 2$).

5.6 Conclusions

NT may serve to confirm or not the clinical suspect of a neurological dysfunction after RP/UD since false-positive findings are very rare; this is especially useful when clinical findings are not completely consistent or for prognostic and therapeutic purposes. Moreover, NT may clarify the pathophysiology of perineal disturbances post RP. Timing of NT is not established, but it is likely that ≥1 month after surgery is necessary to establish whether there has been axonal damage and its severity. Longitudinal follow-up may serve to monitor whether there is spontaneous recovery over time. Controlled prospective studies that include clinical outcome measures and long-term follow-up outcomes would be useful to ascertain the reliability and prognostic value of NT. Since the site of neurological damage is often known a priori in view of the postsurgical onset, the purpose of NT in this setting is to establish the type and severity of involvement, and possibly the side with more severe involvement (if an asymmetry is present, which cannot be ascertained clinically), which may turn useful in terms of pharmacological/rehabilitative intervention, prognosis, and, possibly, prediction of outcome after sacral neuromodulation.

References

1. Han JH, Ku JH. Robot-assisted radical cystectomy: where we are in 2023. Investig Clin Urol. 2023;64(2):107–17. https://doi.org/10.4111/icu.20220384.
2. Marra G, Marquis A, Yanagisawa T, Shariat SF, Touijer K, Gontero P. Salvage radical prostatectomy for recurrent prostate cancer after primary nonsurgical treatment: an updated systematic review. Eur Urol Focus. 2023;9(2):251–7. https://doi.org/10.1016/j.euf.2023.01.013.
3. Territo A, Baboudjian M, Diana P, Gallioli A, Verri P, Uleri A, Basile G, Tedde A, Gaya JM, Huguet J, Rodriguez-Faba O, Sanguedolce F, Sanz Gomez I, Sanchez Molina R, Palou J, Breda A. To drain or not to drain in uro-oncological robotic surgery? A systematic review and meta-analysis. Minerva Urol Nephrol. 2023;75(2):144–53. https://doi.org/10.23736/S2724-6051.22.05160-6.
4. Klovning A, Avery K, Sandvik H, Hunskaar S. Comparison of two questionnaires for assessing the severity of urinary incontinence: the ICIQ-UI SF versus the incontinence severity index. Neurourol Urodyn. 2009;28(5):411–5. https://doi.org/10.1002/nau.20674.
5. Rosen RC, Cappelleri JC, Gendrano N 3rd. The International Index of Erectile Function (IIEF): a state-of-the-science review. Int J Impot Res. 2002;14(4):226–44. https://doi.org/10.1038/sj.ijir.3900857.
6. Bianchi F, Squintani GM, Osio M, Morini A, Bana C, Ardolino G, Barbieri S, Bertolasi L, Caramelli R, Cogiamanian F, Currà A, de Scisciolo G, Foresti C, Frasca V, Frasson E, Inghilleri M, Maderna L, Motti L, Onesti E, Romano MC, Del Carro U. Neurophysiology of the pelvic floor in clinical practice: a systematic literature review. Funct Neurol. 2017;22(4):173–93. https://doi.org/10.11138/fneur/2017.32.4.173.
7. Tankisi H, Pugdahl K, Rasmussen MM, Clemmensen D, Rawashdeh YF, Christensen P, Krogh K, Fuglsang-Frederiksen A. Pelvic floor electrophysiology in spinal cord injury. Clin Neurophysiol. 2016;127(5):2319–24. https://doi.org/10.1016/j.clinph.2015.12.022.
8. Vodusek DB, Fowler CJ, Deletis V, Podnar S. Clinical neurophysiology of pelvic floor disorders. Suppl Clin Neurophysiol. 2000;53:220–7. https://doi.org/10.1016/s1567-424x(09)70162-x.
9. Kiff ES, Swash M. Slowed conduction in the pudendal nerves in idiopathic (neurogenic) faecal incontinence. Br J Surg. 1984;71(8):614–6. https://doi.org/10.1002/bjs.1800710817.
10. Rubin DI. Needle electromyography: basic concepts. Handb Clin Neurol. 2019;160:243–56. https://doi.org/10.1016/B978-0-444-64032-1.00016-3.
11. Kwok WY, So BCL, Ng SMS. Underwater surface electromyography for the evaluation of muscle activity during front crawl swimming: a systematic review. J Sports Sci Med. 2023;22(1):1–16. https://doi.org/10.52082/jssm.2023.1.
12. Giuliano F, Rowland DL. Standard operating procedures for neurophysiologic assessment of male sexual dysfunction. J Sex Med. 2013;10(5):1205–11. https://doi.org/10.1111/jsm.12164.
13. Graves DE. Bulbocavernosus or anal reflex, one or both should be tested after spinal cord injury. Spinal Cord Ser Cases. 2020;6:4. https://doi.org/10.1038/s41394-019-0253-1.
14. Schmid DM, Curt A, Hauri D, Schurch B. Clinical value of combined electrophysiological and urodynamic recordings to assess sexual disorders in spinal cord injured men. Neurourol Urodyn. 2003;22(4):314–21. https://doi.org/10.1002/nau.10125.
15. Catarin MV, Manzano GM, Nóbrega JA, Almeida FG, Srougi M, Bruschini H. The role of membranous urethral afferent autonomic innervation in the continence mechanism after nerve sparing radical prostatectomy: a clinical and prospective study. J Urol. 2008;180(6):2527–31. https://doi.org/10.1016/j.juro.2008.08.020.
16. Gerbaud F, Charlanes A, Chesnel C, Voiry C, Le Breton F, Amarenco G, Manceau P. Effect of radical prostatectomy on involuntary pelvic floor muscle contraction. Neurourol Urodyn. 2019;38(4):1093–9. https://doi.org/10.1002/nau.23959.

17. Hacad CR, Glazer HI, Zambon JP, Burti JS, Almeida FG. Is there any change in pelvic floor electromyography during the first 6 months after radical retropubic prostatectomy? Appl Psychophysiol Biofeedback. 2015;40(1):9–15. https://doi.org/10.1007/s10484-015-9271-3.
18. Shefi S, Zwecker M, Pinthus JH, Mor Y, Zeilig G, Shemesh Y, Hanani JI, Raviv G. Bulbocavernosus reflex testing: a preliminary study on the prognostic factors for potency and response to sildenafil citrate after bilateral nerve-sparing radical prostatectomy. Int Urol Nephrol. 2010;42(1):39–45. https://doi.org/10.1007/s11255-009-9581-6.
19. Turmel N, Ismael SS, Chesnel C, Charlanes A, Hentzen C, Le Breton F, Amarenco G. Use of a specific questionnaire and perineal electromyography to assess neuropathic pain after radical retropubic prostatectomy. Asian J Urol. 2019;6(4):364–7. https://doi.org/10.1016/j.ajur.2018.06.004.
20. Ventimiglia B, Sigona M, Di Dio A, Puglisi T, Costantino G. Urinary incontinence and neuropathy after radical prostatectomy: diagnosis and treatment. Urol J. 2015;82(1):42–5. https://doi.org/10.5301/uro.5000064.
21. Yildiz A, Islamoglu E, Yuksel M, Erol I, Karamik K, Cakir T, Ates M, Savas M. Assessment of changes in penile sensation by electrophysiological study after radical prostatectomy: a pilot study. Curr Urol. 2021;15(2):111–4. https://doi.org/10.1097/CU9.0000000000000016.
22. Zermann DH, Ishigooka M, Wunderlich H, Reichelt O, Schubert J. A study of pelvic floor function pre- and postradical prostatectomy using clinical neurourological investigations, urodynamics and electromyography. Eur Urol. 2000;37(1):72–8. https://doi.org/10.1159/000020103.
23. Yiou R, De Laet K, Hisano M, Salomon L, Abbou CC, Lefaucheur JP. Neurophysiological testing to assess penile sensory nerve damage after radical prostatectomy. J Sex Med. 2012;9(9):2457–66. https://doi.org/10.1111/j.1743-6109.2012.02793.x.
24. Panebianco V, Barchetti F, Sciarra A, Marcantonio A, Zini C, Salciccia S, Collettini F, Gentile V, Hamm B, Catalano C. In vivo 3D neuroanatomical evaluation of periprostatic nerve plexus with 3T-MR diffusion tensor imaging. Eur J Radiol. 2013;82(10):1677–82. https://doi.org/10.1016/j.ejrad.2013.05.013.
25. De Wachter S, Vaganee D, Kessler TM. Sacral neuromodulation: mechanism of action. Eur Urol Focus. 2020;6(5):823–5. https://doi.org/10.1016/j.euf.2019.11.018.
26. Sampogna G, Montanari E, Spinelli M. Computer-assisted lead placement for peripheral nerve evaluation test in a candidate for sacral neuromodulation. Int Neurourol J. 2020;24(4):382–6. https://doi.org/10.5213/inj.2040096.048.
27. Spinelli M, Malaguti S, Giardiello G, Lazzeri M, Tarantola J, Van Den Hombergh U. A new minimally invasive procedure for pudendal nerve stimulation to treat neurogenic bladder: description of the method and preliminary data. Neurourol Urodyn. 2005;24(4):305–9.

6 Pharmacological Therapies for Urinary, Bowel, and Erectile Dysfunction

Maria Angela Cerruto, Paola Irene Ornaghi, Yazan Al Salhi, and Antonio Luigi Pastore

6.1 Pharmacological Therapies for Urinary Dysfunction

Urination or micturition removes metabolic products and toxic wastes filtered from the kidneys and is a vital function of the human body. The micturition reflex requires a complex network of signals between the nervous and urinary tract systems. Urine storage and emptying are highly dependent on these pathways. For these reasons, neurological function and anatomic abnormalities can involve many disease states such as incontinence, obstruction, or infections [1].

6.1.1 Physiology of Urination

The function of the lower urinary tract is characterized by the periodic succession of filling and emptying phases. The filling phase accounts for 98% of the urinary cycle, and when a correct urinary volume is collected, the anatomical functional unit of the lower urinary tract ensures rapid and complete bladder emptying by converting the continuous urinary excretion of the kidneys into an intermittent release process [1].

M. A. Cerruto (✉) · P. I. Ornaghi
Urology Clinic, Department of Surgery, Dentistry, Paediatrics and Gynaecology, University of Verona, Verona, Italy
e-mail: mariaangela.cerruto@univr.it

Y. Al Salhi · A. L. Pastore
Urology Clinic, Department of Medico Surgical Sciences and Biotechnologies, Sapienza University of Rome, Latina, Italy
e-mail: yazan.alsalhi@uniroma1.it; antonioluigi.pastore@uniroma1.it

G. Lamberti, C. De Nunzio (eds.), *Bladder, Bowel and Sexual Dysfunctions Rehabilitation after Radical Prostatectomy*, Urodynamics, Neurourology and Pelvic Floor Dysfunctions, https://doi.org/10.1007/978-3-031-76341-0_6

The anatomical functional unit of the lower urinary tract is represented by the bladder and bladder neck, urethra and urethral sphincter, and pelvic floor [2]. The physiological succession of filling and emptying phases is ensured by the presence of a basic neurological control mechanism that interacts with a pattern of related activities associated with numerous social, environmental, and behavioral factors. Urination, as the end product of this complex process, requires careful neurological control involving the central nervous system and the peripheral nervous system, both autonomic and somatic.

Due to the complexity of central nervous control of the lower urinary tract, urinary urge incontinence can develop as a result of various conditions such as aging, certain neurological diseases, urinary disorders, and bladder myogenic changes, which are responsible for the onset of detrusor overactivity (DO).

When the anatomical functional unit of the lower urinary tract is unable to function properly or there is a loss of balance between the complex neurological control mechanisms, urinary dysfunction occurs, which may primarily involve the filling phase, the emptying phase, or both.

Aging, neurological diseases, and certain diseases of the lower urinary tract can alter the voluntary control of urination, causing the re-emergence of involuntary reflex mechanisms present in childhood and responsible for the onset of DO and urge urinary incontinence (UUI) [3]. Pharmacotherapy aims to restore normal voluntary urinary control by inhibiting emerging pathological reflex circuits.

Many drugs have been proposed according to possible therapeutic targets, both central and peripheral, but the results are often disappointing partly due to poor therapeutic efficacy and partly to side effects. The development of pharmacological treatment of different forms of urinary incontinence is slow and the use of some of the drugs currently prescribed and on the market is based more on tradition than on evidence derived from controlled clinical trials.

6.1.2 Overactive Bladder and DO

Overactive bladder (OAB) is a common clinical entity that affects both men and women. It is highly prevalent, and rates generally increase with advancing age, making it even more common in older and frail older adults. OAB is a symptoms syndrome characterized by "urgency, with or without urge urinary incontinence, usually with frequency and nocturia … if there is no proven infection or other obvious pathology" [4]. This combination of symptoms is suggestive of urodynamically demonstrable DO, defined as "a urodynamic observation characterized by involuntary detrusor contractions during the filling phase" [4].

OAB is not a synonym of DO and vice versa: DO is only detected in about half of patients with OAB by conventional technique and, on the other hand, up to 50% of patients having DO did not complain of relevant clinical symptoms [5]. The only currently available tool to link them is urodynamics. Nevertheless, they share therapeutic options and, partially, a virtual common underlying physiopathological mechanism [5].

The main aim of pharmacotherapy is to restore normal control of micturition, inhibiting the emerging pathological involuntary reflex mechanism. Therapeutic targets can be identified in the urothelium, detrusor muscles, autonomic and afferent pathways, spinal cord, and brain [6]. Increased expression and/or sensitivity of urothelial sensory molecules that lead to afferent sensitization have been documented as a possible pathogenesis of OAB. Targeting afferent pathways and/or bladder smooth muscles by modulating the activity of ligand receptors and ion channels could be effective to suppress OAB [6].

Currently, antimuscarinics represent the first-line treatment in cases of OAB [5, 7, 8]. When antimuscarinic therapy fails, other drugs for facilitation of urine storage can be used like mixed-action drugs, drugs acting on cell membrane channels, alpha-adrenergic antagonists, beta-adrenergic agonists, inhibitors of prostaglandin synthesis, and other drugs (antidepressants, desmopressin, estrogens, muscle relaxants, capsaicin, botulinum toxin).

6.1.2.1 Antimuscarinic Drugs

The rationale for antimuscarinic therapy in the treatment of UUI is based on the blocking of muscarinic receptors (MRs) at both detrusor and non-detrusor sites to prevent symptoms of OAB and DO without suppressing detrusor contraction during bladder emptying; reduce episodes of urgency and urge incontinence; increase bladder capacity; and reduce the number of urinations per day, to achieve an overall improvement in the patient's quality of life [9].

Most antimuscarinic drugs lack selectivity for bladder receptors causing several side effects that are sometimes intolerable for the patient. The occurrence of systemic side effects by antimuscarinics is justified by the wide distribution of muscarinic receptors in different body districts.

Depending on the different target organ, the following side effects may occur: blurred vision due to defect of accommodation, dry eyes due to blockage of the lacrimal glands, dry mouth due to blockage of the salivary glands, poor digestion due to reduced production of hydrochloric acid, and constipation [10, 11].

In addition, sensitivity to antimuscarinic side effects increases with age, particularly concerning the central nervous system, accentuating memory disturbances, drowsiness, and mental confusion [12, 13]. Generally, an individual titration of the antimuscarinic used is advisable to achieve the maximum effect with the least possible side effects, although some authors argue that higher doses of drugs may be needed in patients over 75 years of age [14, 15]. Contraindications to the use of antimuscarinics include narrow-angle glaucoma and cervico-urethral obstruction (the latter due to the potential risk of urinary retention).

There is a higher prevalence of comorbidity among the elderly, which can further reduce treatment efficacy and heighten the potential for side effects to occur. Failure to acknowledge the multifactorial nature of urinary incontinence in the elderly often leads to suboptimal treatment. Urgency symptoms may be exacerbated by the consumption of caffeinated beverages, pelvic floor muscle weakness, diuretics, or other functional and systemic dysfunctions. Treatment should therefore address all possible etiologies and not be limited to a solitary intervention. Combining behavioral and drug therapy yields greater improvements in OAB symptoms than drug therapy alone but not behavioral therapy alone. Burgio et al. suggested that when using a stepped approach, it is reasonable to begin with behavioral therapy alone [16, 17].

A growing body of literature has emerged to address the concern that antimuscarinic agents used to treat symptoms of overactive bladder may cross the blood-brain barrier, bind to muscarinic receptors within the central nervous system (CNS), and provoke subtle or not so subtle cognitive impairment, especially in older elderly people [18, 19].

As already described in the review article by Pagoria et al., and confirmed in the work by Welk et al. published in Nature Reviews Urology [20], the trials that have performed cognitive testing in healthy elderly people taking antimuscarinics have clearly shown that oxybutynin can adversely affect cognition; meanwhile, darifenacin, trospium, solifenacin, and tolterodine have not shown such substantial effects on short-term cognitive function. Moreover, the integrity of the blood-brain barrier may be compromised in many older adults with cerebrovascular disease, diabetes, or certain forms of dementia. Therefore, especially in elderly patients with potential risk factors for cognitive impairment or preexisting dementia [21], the cautious use of selected OAB anticholinergic agents with favorable physicochemical and pharmacokinetic properties and clinical trial evidence of cognitive safety might be appropriate [20].

In addition to the impact of prolonged use of antimuscarinic drugs for OAB, it should also be taken into account that many commonly prescribed medications in the elderly possess antimuscarinic properties [22], so the results may not be specific to bladder antimuscarinics [23–25]. Other antimuscarinic medications include, among others, amitriptyline, clozapine, olanzapine, paroxetine, furosemide, hydrocodone, lansoprazole, levofloxacin, and metformin.

The main antimuscarinic drugs used in OAB are listed below (oxybutynin will be discussed later as a mixed-action drug).

Atropine	Rarely used for the treatment of UUI but may maintain a role in the intravesical treatment of patients with neurogenic DO and urination problems requiring intermittent catheterization such as those with multiple sclerosis [26, 27]
Solifenacin	Used to reduce urgency, UUI, and urinary frequency by improving bladder capacity. It has low rates of both dry mouth and discontinuation of therapy due to the occurrence of adverse events
Trospium chloride	Documented efficacy comparable to oxybutynin in the treatment of DO [28]. The hydrophilicity and quaternary amine structure of trospium may limit its ability to cross the blood-brain barrier and thus minimize the impact on cognition, especially in the elderly [29, 30]
Fesoterodine	Generally well tolerated even in elderly patients because few drug-to-drug interactions have been demonstrated [29, 31]. Most cases of dry mouth and constipation were mild or moderate, and the discontinuation rates associated with these adverse events did not increase with age [15]
Tolterodine	Significantly improved OAB symptoms and patients' quality of life compared to placebo even if it persists statistically significant advantages for fesoterodine compared with tolterodine [31]. Limited ability to cross the blood-brain barrier, justifying the low incidence of neurological side effects. Functional selectivity in the bladder compared to the salivary glands [28]
Darifenacin	Can significantly reduce the number of UUI episodes, urgency severity, and frequency of urination [28]. Not demonstrated significant adverse effects on the central nervous system and cardiovascular system [32]. Mild to moderate dry mouth and constipation [29]

6.1.2.2 Mixed-Action Drugs

Some drugs used to block DO have been shown to have more than one mechanism of action. They all have a more or less pronounced antimuscarinic effect and, in addition, an often poorly defined "direct" action on bladder muscle. For many of these drugs, the antimuscarinic effect manifests itself at concentrations considerably lower than those useful for causing a "direct" bladder response that would involve blocking voltage-dependent calcium channels. Thus, the clinical effect of such mixed-action drugs can be explained mainly by their antimuscarinic action [8].

Oxybutynin chloride	Antimuscarinic, calcium antagonist, and local anesthetic activity. The anesthetic action may be of some importance when the drug is instilled intravesically but not when it is administered orally [33]. When administered orally, it behaves primarily as an antimuscarinic drug. It has a high affinity for bladder muscarinic receptors but also shows philia for muscarinic receptors in the salivary glands. Systemic side effects: dry mouth, blurred vision, constipation, and tachycardia, which frequently occur in patients orally treated [28, 34, 35]. Possible alternative routes of drug administration in addition to the oral and intravesical routes are the transrectal and transdermal routes [28, 29, 35]
Propiverine hydrochloride	Both antimuscarinic and calcium antagonist action. Effective in the decrease in the number of micturitions/day, urgencies, urgency incontinence, and nocturia and increases urine volume [36]. In idiopathic DO demonstrated similar efficacy to that of other antimuscarinic agents and, in adults with neurogenic DO, demonstrated similar efficacy of oxybutynin [37]. The major adverse event reported is difficulty in voiding. Combining it with an alpha1-adrenoceptor antagonist was more effective in terms of decreasing difficulty in voiding [36, 37]
Flavoxate hydrochloride	No anticholinergic effect. Moderate calcium antagonist action; inhibiting action on phosphodiesterase; local anesthetic properties. Widely used and accepted among urologists and general physicians for decades globally [38]. Flavoxate can be considered effective and well tolerated, with almost negligible side effects, making it worthy of consideration for the treatment of OAB [39]

6.1.2.3 Alpha-Adrenergic Antagonist

Alpha-adrenergic antagonists (tamsulosin, alfuzosin, terazosin, doxazosin, and silodosin), typically used clinically for managing outlet obstruction symptoms in men, can reduce the frequency and amplitude of non-voiding contractions in rats with partial bladder outlet obstruction [40]. The rationale for the use of alpha-adrenergic antagonists in OAB is based on the observation that alpha-adrenergic antagonists can improve urinary symptoms in men with benign prostatic hypertrophy and may occasionally abolish the DO present in this category of patients [41]. Alpha1-blockers and antimuscarinic agents registered an additive ameliorative effect on DO when co-administered at low doses: alpha1-blockers prevent the reduction in bladder contraction duration induced by a high-dose administration of antimuscarinic agents [42].

6.1.2.4 Beta-Adrenergic Agonists

Unsatisfactory clinical effectiveness and suboptimal tolerance of cholinolytics have become an impulse to seek new drugs for OAB [43]. In the isolated human bladder, non-subtype-selective beta-adrenergic agonists have a pronounced inhibitory effect on detrusor contractility, justifying their possible clinical use. These medications offer a theoretical advantage by avoiding anticholinergic effects associated with most antimuscarinic medications that could potentially be problematic in geriatric patients [44, 45].

Mirabegron	Demonstrated significant efficacy in treating symptoms of OAB and significant improvements versus placebo [46]. Specifically comparing elderly and younger subjects, the β-3 agonist mirabegron appeared to be safe and effective [44, 45]. Like darifenacin, mirabegron was found to be a drug that, in the short term, does not adversely affect cognitive function even in patients with a history of a cerebrovascular accident [32, 47]
Vibegron	Provided statistically significant reductions in micturitions, urgency episodes, and urge incontinence and increased the volume per micturition [48]. Less likely to cause drug-drug interaction compared to mirabegron. Moreover, since this drug does not penetrate the blood-brain barrier, it could become the drug of choice in OAB patients with cognitive impairment [43]

6.1.2.5 Prostaglandin Synthesis Inhibitors

Some mechanisms have been proposed to modulate afferent activity in the lower urinary tract. Several substances, including neurotrophins, prostaglandins, and tachykinins, may contribute to altered afferent excitability [6, 49]. Prostaglandins are involved in the micturition reflex in rats mainly mediated by the cyclooxygenase (COX)-2 isozyme: Benefits of nonsteroidal anti-inflammatory drugs have been reported clinically, but this approach has not become standard practice because of doubts about the efficacy and high incidence of adverse effects [50]. Nonetheless, interest in prostaglandins is likely to increase again now that their participation in cellular interactions in the bladder wall has been described [51]. Recent studies present prostaglandin receptor systems as a potential regulator of urinary bladder contractility: The urinary bladder urothelium with lamina propria and detrusor smooth muscle respond to an analog variety of prostaglandin agonists, with their activation resulting in direct contractions, as well as increases to spontaneous contractile activity [52, 53]. It follows that treatment with prostaglandin synthesis inhibitors might be effective in inhibiting involuntary detrusor contractions. Unfortunately, the few controlled clinical trials on the effects of such drugs in the treatment of DO and the number of drugs tested make it difficult to appropriately assess the therapeutic value of prostaglandin synthesis inhibitors.

6.1.2.6 Other Treatments

5α-reductase inhibitors	For the treatment of lower urinary tract symptoms suggestive of benign prostatic hyperplasia ("LUTS/BPH") with large prostate (prostate volume > 30 mL), the combination of an α-blocker and a 5α-reductase inhibitor (dutasteride/finasteride) has been reported to be more effective, even in the storage symptoms, compared to each monotherapy [54, 55]. However, the combination of α-blocker, dutasteride, and the anticholinergic drug has been reported to be more effective than the combination of α-blocker plus dutasteride for the treatment of "BPH/OAB" with large prostate (DIrecT study) [56, 57]
Phosphodiesterase-5 inhibitors	Phosphodiesterase (PDE)-5 inhibitors have been recently recommended as monotherapy for BPH/LUTS [58–61]. Furthermore, tadalafil add-on therapy was not inferior to solifenacin add-on therapy in terms of effect and safety as an alternative add-on drug for patients with persistent lower urinary tract symptoms refractory to α1-adrenoceptor antagonists [62]. The effect of tadalafil/mirabegron combination therapy on relieving OAB symptoms appeared to be greater than that of tadalafil monotherapy and can be safely used [63]
Antidepressants	Reported positive effects on the therapeutic management of patients with DO. Tricyclic antidepressants, such as imipramine, inhibit the micturition reflex in rats but through a mechanism unrelated to any antimuscarinic effect [64, 65]. Numerically few studies have been conducted and no RCT of good quality has documented the efficacy of imipramine in the treatment of DO. However, a beneficial effect has been documented in the treatment of nocturnal enuresis
Desmopressin	Most frequently tested medication for the specific treatment of nocturia (traditionally been used to treat primary nocturnal enuresis and nocturnal polyuria in adults) [66]. Efficacious in significantly reducing nighttime urine production, episodes of nocturia, and urgency episodes [67]. Relevant effectivity of the combination therapy with anticholinergic drugs with least side effects for the treatment of OAB/nocturnal polyuria [67, 68]. Most frequently adverse events include headache, hyponatremia, insomnia, dry mouth, hypertension, abdominal pain, peripheral edema, and nausea [69]. Although side effects are infrequent, there is a risk of water retention and hyponatremia; therefore, in the elderly, it must be used with caution
Capsaicin	Instilled into the bladder, it has been shown to be effective in the treatment of neurogenic DO but is burdened by side effects that limit its use. Resiniferatoxin (RTX) is an ultra-potent analog of capsaicin extracted from Euphorbia resinifera. Administered intravesically, it has been shown to be as effective as capsaicin in the treatment of neurogenic DO but much less irritating [70]. Currently, the use of vanilloids cannot be recommended for routine use in patients with OAB as the need for catheterization may cause the risk to outweigh the benefit of treatment [71]

Botulinum toxin A	Produced by the Gram+ bacterium Clostridium botulinum and is capable of selectively blocking the release of acetylcholine from nerve endings and has been used as a second-line treatment of neurogenic DO [72]. Botulinum toxin (at a dose of 200–300 units in patients with neurogenic DO and 100–200 units in those with idiopathic DO) is injected endoscopically into the detrusor muscle at 20–30 different sites, sparing the trigone. Botox selectively disrupts and modulates neurotransmission, suppresses detrusor overactivity, and modulates sensory function, inflammation, and glandular function. In addition to motor effects, Botox has been found to have sensory inhibitory effects and anti-inflammatory effects; therefore, it has been tested to treat interstitial cystitis/bladder pain syndrome (IC/BPS) [73, 74]. However, the use of Botox for IC/BPS has not been approved. Adverse events included urinary tract infection, pain at the injection site, hematuria, and autonomic dysreflexia [72]

6.1.3 Stress Urinary Incontinence

The International Continence Society defines stress urinary incontinence (SUI) as the complaint of involuntary leakage on effort, exertion, sneezing, or coughing [75]. SUI is a symptom mainly caused by sphincteric incompetence and usually occurs in women after delivery or pelvic surgery, whereas most cases of male UI occur after radical prostatectomy (RP). UI after RP is related to the lack of urethral support and intrinsic sphincter deficiency in most patients although DO or abnormalities in bladder neck function may also exist [76].

Pharmacological treatment of stress urinary incontinence aims to increase endourethral pressure either by increasing the tone of the urethral smooth muscle or by acting on the striated muscles at both the urethral and pelvic floor sites. Several drugs have been proposed for this purpose: alpha-adrenergic agonists, beta-adrenergic antagonists, clenbuterol, serotonin, and noradrenaline reuptake inhibitors such as imipramine and duloxetine.

Alpha-adrenergic agonists	May increase urethral resistance by modifying urethral pressure. Effective in increasing bladder outlet resistance during bladder filling in animal models [77]. Alpha-adrenoceptor agonists lack exclusive selectivity for urethral a-adrenoceptors and may cause severe systemic side effects such as elevated blood pressure, sleep disturbances, nausea, dry mouth, headache, tremor, palpitations, and exacerbation of abnormal cardiac rhythms [5]. Although the use of propranolol has shown positive effects in the treatment of stress urinary incontinence, there are currently no RCTs supporting its use
Beta2-adrenoceptor agonist	Clenbuterol, a bronchodilator for patients with asthma, has been shown to be potentially useful in the management of male SUI. Adverse effects of clenbuterol are reported to be tremors, tachycardia, arrhythmia, increased sweating, and headache. However, it has not been rigorously tested in clinical trials yet and, therefore, has not received approval for the treatment of SUI by the FDA or the European Agency for the Evaluation of Medical Products (EMEA) [76]

Duloxetine	Among men with postprostatectomy SUI or mixed urinary incontinence (stress predominant), who were randomized to duloxetine and placebo at least 1 year after surgery, there was a 50–100% decrease in incontinence episode frequency (IEF) at 12 weeks in over half of the patients [78]. Duloxetine has demonstrated good short-term cure and/or improvement in treating men with persistent post-RP SUI, as well as in reducing the time to attain continence [79]. The most common adverse events (>5%) include nausea, fatigue, insomnia, dry mouth, constipation, dizziness, and headache [61]

Promising new studies are focusing on the therapy of post-RP SUI using a periurethral injection of autologous adipose-derived regenerative cells [80]. These studies suggest the efficacy and safety of regenerative treatment for male patients with mild-to-moderate stress urinary incontinence [81], especially in younger patients (<70 years) [82].

6.1.4 Urinary Incontinence in Patients with Chronic Urine Retention

Urinary retention is the acute or chronic inability to voluntarily pass an adequate amount of urine. The condition predominantly affects men and excludes transient micturition difficulties (e.g., after anti-incontinence surgery). The most common causes are obstructive in nature, with benign prostatic hyperplasia accounting for 53% of cases. Infectious, inflammatory, iatrogenic, and neurologic causes can also affect urinary retention. The initial evaluation should involve a detailed history that includes information about current prescription medications and the use of over-the-counter medications and herbal supplements. A focused physical examination with neurologic evaluation should be performed, and diagnostic testing should include measurement of postvoid residual (PVR) volume of urine. The American Urological Association recommends that chronic urinary retention be defined as PVR volume greater than 300 mL measured on two separate occasions and persisting for at least 6 months [83].

Initial management of urinary retention involves assessment of urethral patency with prompt and complete bladder decompression by catheterization, and further management is decided by determining the cause and chronicity of the urinary retention. The pharmacological treatment of urinary incontinence secondary to chronic urinary retention aims to prevent upper urinary tract damage by normalizing bladder emptying and endourethral pressures. The drugs that have been used for this purpose are alpha-adrenergic antagonists, muscarinic receptor agonists, and anticholinesterases for their parasympathetic-mimetic effect, intravesical prostaglandins, baclofen, benzodiazepines, and dantrolene.

Muscarinic receptor agonists, anticholinesterases, and beta-adrenergic antagonists have not been shown to be effective in significantly increasing intravesical pressure, thereby promoting bladder emptying. Stimulation of detrusor activity with intravesical instillations of prostaglandins has been reported to be effective, although the results are controversial, and no randomized clinical trials are available [84]. Alpha-adrenergic antagonists may have a role in reducing urethral resistance, especially in initial management, added to voiding trials, but RCTs are lacking and current evidence is inconsistent [83, 85].

Baclofen, benzodiazepines, and dantrolene are reported to play a role in reducing flow resistance in particular categories of patients with chronic urinary retention secondary to muscle spasticity. Even for these drugs, there are no RCTs supporting their possible use [86]. Phenoxybenzamine (PBZ) is no longer used in clinical trials due to its possible carcinogenic effects and side effects even if no drug-related tumors in humans have been reported after −50 years of clinical experience with PBZ and clinical trials have demonstrated that it can relieve symptoms in patients with BPH and other urologic and pain-related conditions [87].

6.2 Pharmacological Therapies for Bowel Dysfunction

6.2.1 Chronic Constipation

Chronic constipation is a common, persistent condition affecting many patients worldwide, presenting significant economic burdens and resulting in substantial healthcare utilization. In addition to infrequent bowel movements, the definition of constipation includes excessive straining, a sense of incomplete evacuation, failed or lengthy attempts to defecate, use of digital maneuvers for evacuation of stool, abdominal bloating, and hard consistency of stools. Clinical assessment of the patient with constipation requires careful history taking to identify any red flag symptoms that would necessitate further investigation with colonoscopy to exclude colorectal malignancy. Screening for hypercalcemia, hypothyroidism, and celiac disease with appropriate blood tests should be considered [88].

After excluding secondary causes of constipation, chronic idiopathic or primary constipation can be classified as functional defecation disorder, slow-transit constipation (STC), and constipation-predominant irritable bowel syndrome (IBS-C) [89–91]. These classifications are not mutually exclusive and significant overlap exists.

The initial therapeutic approach to primary constipation, regardless of etiology, consists of diet and lifestyle changes such as encouraging adequate fluid and fiber intake, regular exercise, and dietary modification. Laxatives are the mainstay of pharmacological treatment for potential long-term therapy in patients who do not respond to lifestyle or dietary modification. After a failed empiric trial of laxatives, diagnostic testing is necessary to understand underlying anorectal and/or colonic pathophysiology. No single test provides a comprehensive assessment for primary constipation; therefore, multiple tests are used to provide complementary information to one another [92].

Patients not responding to traditional laxatives should be offered treatment with prosecretory agents such as lubiprostone, linaclotide, and plecanatide or the 5-HT4 receptor agonist prucalopride, where available. If there is no response to pharmacological treatment, surgical intervention can be considered, but it is only suitable for a carefully selected subset of patients with proven slow-transit constipation [88].

A digital rectal examination should be performed to assess for evidence of dyssynergic defecation. If this is suspected, further investigation with high-resolution anorectal manometry should be undertaken. Anorectal biofeedback can be offered to patients with dyssynergic defecation as a means of correcting the associated impairment of the pelvic floor, abdominal wall, and rectal functioning [88]. Dyssynergic defecation, a functional defecation disorder, is an acquired behavioral disorder of defecation present in two-thirds of adult patients, where an inability to coordinate the abdominal, recto-anal, and pelvic floor muscles during attempted defecation exists [93]. Biofeedback therapy is the mainstay treatment for dyssynergic defecation aimed at improving the coordination of abdominal and anorectal muscles. A large percentage of patients with dyssynergic defecation also exhibit rectal hyposensitivity and may benefit from the addition of sensory retraining [94].

The advent of high-resolution colonic manometry (HRCM) allows for the improved identification of colonic motor patterns and may provide further insight into pathophysiological mechanisms. Recently, HRCM has rapidly developed into a major technique for obtaining more effective information involved in the physiology and/or pathophysiology of colonic contractile activity in colonic dysmotility patients [95]. In a minority of cases of STC, identification of colonic neuropathy suggests a medically refractory condition, warranting consideration of colectomy. Colonic microbiota may also play a role in the pathophysiology of STC. Regulating the intestinal environment may be a novel therapeutic strategy for constipation [96].

The pathophysiology of IBS-C is poorly understood with multiple etiological factors implicated. Pharmacological advances in the treatment of primary constipation have added therapeutic options to the armamentarium of this disorder [97]. Drug development in the secretagogue, serotonergic prokinetic, and ileal bile acid transporter inhibition pathways has yielded current and future medical treatment options for primary chronic constipation [92].

6.2.2 Fecal Incontinence

Fecal incontinence is a devastating disease for those whom it affects. Although no consensus definition exists, it is generally accepted that accidental leakage of liquid or solid stool for more than 1 month is required to make the diagnosis [98]. The disorder is common, and prevalence varies depending on the population studied. Among institutionalized persons, the prevalence has been reported as high as 45% [99]. The personal and financial burden is huge, with the majority of cases remaining undiagnosed and hence not treated [100]. Several pathophysiological mechanisms have been identified and include advancing age, parity, pelvic floor dysfunction, stool form disturbance, and chronic obstructive airways disease [101]. The relative lack of efficacy of many established treatments further highlights the need to uncover contributing causes and hence better future therapeutic targets.

Conservative medical management consisting of patient education, fiber supplements or antidiarrheals, behavioral techniques such as scheduled toileting, and pelvic floor exercises restores continence in up to 25% of patients [102].

After a specific diagnosis is established, appropriate therapy can be commenced. Treatment of fecal incontinence associated with diarrhea will be very different from that of patients with leakage associated with fecal impaction (pseudo-diarrhea), highlighting the need to address any underlying cause when possible. Antidiarrheals such as loperamide have an established role in chronic diarrhea of any cause, but their use is often limited by constipation [103].

Amitriptyline has modest efficacy for symptoms in patients with idiopathic fecal incontinence [104]. Recent developments in medical therapy include trials of transdermal clonidine. Promising results from a recent open-label study by Bharucha et al. [105] showed clonidine increased the number of incontinence-free days and reduced the fecal incontinence symptoms scores in women with predominantly urge-pattern fecal incontinence. Although a larger controlled study is required to validate these findings, this raises the possibility that by addressing abnormalities in anorectal sensorimotor dysfunction, improved continence can be achieved.

Biofeedback therapy aims at retraining the pelvic floor and abdominal wall musculature. Cognitively able patients can gain improved coordination and control of these muscle groups with the aid of an instructing therapist and electromyographic surface electrodes placed on the abdomen and in the rectum [106]. Biofeedback, often recommended as a first-line treatment after conservative management fails, produces satisfaction with treatment in up to 76% and continence in 55%; however, outcomes depend on the skill of the therapist, and some trials are less favorable [102]. Although biofeedback treatment is recommended by several authorities, including the American Gastroenterological Association, convincing evidence of its superiority compared with conservative treatment is lacking as concluded in a Cochrane review [106].

Electrical stimulation of the anal mucosa is ineffective, but the continuous electrical pulsing of sacral nerves produces a ≥50% reduction in fecal incontinence frequency in a median of 73% of patients. Tibial nerve electrical stimulation with needle electrodes is promising but remains unproven [102].

6.2.3 Irritable Bowel Syndrome

Irritable bowel syndrome (IBS) is a chronic and debilitating functional gastrointestinal disorder that presents with abdominal pain associated with the alteration of bowel habits [107]. IBS is a common condition affecting 9–23% of the general population, 80% female, with a considerable impact on quality of life and healthcare costs [108]. The exact pathogenesis of IBS remains elusive but is clearly multifactorial and includes environmental and host factors.

According to the updated ROME III criteria, IBS is a clinical diagnosis and presents as one of the three predominant subtypes: (1) IBS with constipation (IBS-C), (2) IBS with diarrhea (IBS-D), and (3) mixed IBS (IBS-M). Former ROME definitions refer to IBS-M as alternating IBS (IBS-A). Across the IBS subtypes, the presentation of symptoms may vary among patients and change over time. Patients report the most distressing symptoms to be abdominal pain, straining, myalgias, urgency, bloating, and feelings of serious illness [109].

Management of patients with IBS is challenging since diagnosis, treatment could require several approaches with unsatisfactory results, and a personalized approach is needed. In any case, the diagnosis of IBS is based on the positive identification of symptoms consistent with this condition and by excluding an underlying organic disease [107]. A strong, reassuring physician-patient relationship is crucial, followed by patient education, dietary advice, and stress reduction. For nonresponding patients, the therapeutic approach may include nonpharmacological therapies and/or pharmacotherapy [110]. The choice of pharmacological treatment is based on the predominant symptom and a prespecified time point should be planned for effectiveness evaluation and dose adjustment. In patients with IBS-D, the therapeutic options include mainly antibiotics, such as rifaximin, peripheral opioid agonists, mixed opioid agonists/antagonists, bile acid sequestrants, and antagonists of serotonin 5-hydroxytryptamine type 3 receptors. Bulking agents and osmotic laxatives represent the first-line therapy for IBS-C, while lubiprostone and linaclotide should be reserved for difficult-to-treat patients. The involvement of gastrointestinal microbiota constitutes a fascinating field of exploration as it offers the potential to be modulated by the use of probiotics, prebiotics, synbiotics, as well as fecal microbiota transplantation [110].

Erectile dysfunction (ED) is the inability to achieve or maintain an erection sufficient for satisfactory sexual performance [111]. There are several well-recognized risk factors for ED development, including aging, smoking, obesity, diabetes, coronary ischemic disease, peripheral vascular disease, depression, Peyronie's disease, hypertension, and dyslipidemia [2, 112, 113]. Iatrogenic factors include pelvic surgery as well as side effects of medications [112–114]. Medications for ED treatment include oral, injection, and topical therapies [1]. There are new developing treatments that might change the landscape of ED treatment, including next-generation phosphodiesterase type 5 inhibitors (PDE5Is), rho-kinase inhibitors, melanocortin receptor antagonists, nanotechnology, stem cell injection, gene therapy, low-intensity extracorporeal shock wave therapy, and platelet-rich plasma injection.

6.3 Pharmacological Therapies for Erectile Dysfunction

6.3.1 Oral Medications

6.3.1.1 Phosphodiesterase Type 5 Inhibitors

The introduction of the phosphodiesterase type 5 inhibitor (PDE5I) for ED treatment starts with sildenafil citrate in 1998 [111]. Currently, oral PDE5I therapy represents the mainstay first-line treatment of ED and constitutes one of the most prescribed medications for men's health. Tadalafil, vardenafil, and avanafil have all subsequently been approved by the Food and Drug Administration (FDA) [115] and the European Medicines Agency (EMA) [116]. The pharmacokinetics is the principal difference among these drugs, while the efficacy of all PDE5Is has been observed to be similar [117]. Likewise, one key contraindication is in high-risk cardiovascular disease and in patients actively taking nitrate medication [118]. Following sexual stimulus, nitrous oxide (NO) is released by endothelial cells and postsynaptic neurons in the penis. NO enters smooth muscle cells in arterioles and stimulates guanylyl cyclase to convert guanosine triphosphate (GTP) to cyclic guanosine monophosphate (cGMP) [119]. Cyclic GMP triggers a cascade of events that result in arteriolar dilatation and increased blood flow in which combined with veno-occlusion leads to penile erection [115]. Phosphodiesterase type 5 inactivates cGMP, thus reversing the process of tumescence. Inhibition of phosphodiesterase type 5 increases the amount of cGMP in smooth muscle cells, thereby maintaining arteriolar dilatation, increasing rigidity, and prolonging erection [120]. Oral PDE5Is have varying rates of absorption and bioavailability. They are all metabolized by the liver with enzymes CYP3A4, CYP3A5, CYP2C, and CYP2CP predominantly involved [121]. Time to peak serum concentration and clinical effect is known to be delayed by the concurrent ingestion of a fatty meal in all PDE5Is apart from tadalafil [121–123]. Orodispersible PDE5Is tablets (ODT) dissolve within few seconds and can be assumed with or without water [124–127]. Radicioni et al. concluded that the pharmacokinetics of ODT sildenafil did not differ significantly from the existing film-coated version [125]. Vardenafil ODT preparations, however, have demonstrated a better safety profile and bioavailability in comparison with the established film-coated tablet [126]. Regarding PDE5Is efficacy, Goldstein et al. pooled data from 48 double-blinded randomized control trials and 11,364 men with ED. The use of sildenafil was compared to placebo. The percentage of patients reporting improved erectile function decreased with age, with 80% of men under 65 years reporting improvement, 69% of men aged 65–74 falling to 59% of men over 75 [121]. The ENDOTRIAL study compared efficacy of sildenafil, tadalafil, and vardenafil. The outcomes were measured using the self-administered IIEF5 questionnaire as well as penile blood flow parameters studied by echo color Doppler US. The authors concluded that all PDE5Is were similar in terms of erectile function improvement, whereas penile flow improved with an increased dose of sildenafil [122]. Liao et al. conducted a meta-analysis investigating the efficacy of PDE5Is among 5274 diabetic subjects with ED. A mean improvement in IIEF score of 7.1, 8, 9.3, and 5 was observed for sildenafil, vardenafil, mirodenafil, and avanafil, respectively. The authors concluded that vardenafil and mirodenafil were the most advantageous with respect to balancing efficacy while avoiding treatment-related adverse outcomes in this patient population [127]. An earlier meta-analysis conducted in Germany found a mean improvement in IIEF score of 9.7, 8.5, and 7.5 for sildenafil, tadalafil, and vardenafil respectively [128].

6.3.2 Intracavernous Injection

Intracavernous injections (ICI) offer an alternative drug delivery method with a more favorable side effect profile compared to oral pharmacotherapy [129]. The most important advantage of ICI is its efficacy irrespective of an intact nerve supply to the penis (i.e., after non-nerve-sparing radical prostatectomy) [130]. However, given the more invasiveness of injections, ICI remains a second-line option [129]. Moreover, patients must be made aware of the possible side effect, priapism, and the patient must have sufficient manual dexterity to self-administer the injection [131]. Alprostadil is a synthetic prostaglandin E1 (PGE1). It is a vasoactive agent that binds directly to smooth muscle cell prostaglandin receptors, activating adenylate cyclase, which converts ATP to cAMP. This leads to a reduction in intracellular calcium and therefore causes smooth muscle relaxation, cavernosal artery dilatation, increased blood flow, and subsequent erection [132]. Any alprostadil that enters systemic circulation is rapidly metabolized by the lungs and excreted by the kidneys [133]. ICI alprostadil takes clinical effect within 10–15 min and can last up to 12 h [132]. In a meta-analysis of 4577 patients, alprostadil was effective in 70% of patients [134]. However, in a prospective trial examining the completion of intercourse after alprostadil ICI, a success rate of 93% was achieved. Satisfactory sexual experience was reported by 87% of patients and 86% of partners [135]. ICI alprostadil adverse effects have been reported to include prolonged erections in 5%, priapism in 1–4%, fibrosis in 2–8%, hematoma in 8%, and penile pain post injection in 11% [133].

6.3.3 Topical Preparations

Medicated Urethral System for Erection (MUSE©) is a pellet comprising of alprostadil suspended in polyethylene glycol. The medication is delivered via an applicator inserted into the urethra post micturition. There is no recognized risk of priapism or fibrosis, [136]; however, the European Association of Urology (EAU) guidelines report symptoms of penile pain (29–41%), dizziness (1.9–14%), and urethral bleeding (5%) [137]. Erections good enough for intercourse are reported in 30–65.9% of patients [137].

An alternative alprostadil topical agent, Vitaros© cream has been recently introduced and is available in doses of 200 and 300 μg [12]. The cream is applied directly to the glans penis and allowed to absorb for 30 s before any remaining cream is then massaged into the glans. Data on efficacy is limited; however, a recent study of 71 patients observed a mean improvement in IIEF-5 score of 6.3 [138].

References

1. Cortes GA, Flores JL. Physiology, urination. StatPearls [Internet]. Treasure Island (FL): StatPearls Publishing; 2022. http://www.ncbi.nlm.nih.gov/books/NBK562181/. [cited 2022 Nov 15].
2. Hickling DR, Sun T-T, Wu X-R. Anatomy and physiology of the urinary tract: relation to host defense and microbial infection. Microbiol Spectr. 2015;3.
3. de Groat WC, Griffiths D, Yoshimura N. Neural control of the lower urinary tract. Compr Physiol. 2015;5:327–96.
4. Abrams P, Cardozo L, Fall M, Griffiths D, Rosier P, Ulmsten U, et al. The standardisation of terminology in lower urinary tract function: report from the standardisation sub-committee of the International Continence Society. Urology. 2003;61:37–49.
5. Abrams P, Andersson KE, Birder L, Brubaker L, Cardozo L, Chapple C, et al. Fourth International Consultation on Incontinence Recommendations of the International Scientific Committee: evaluation and treatment of urinary incontinence, pelvic organ prolapse, and fecal incontinence. Neurourol Urodyn. 2010;29:213–40.
6. Yoshimura N, Kaiho Y, Miyazato M, Yunoki T, Tai C, Chancellor MB, et al. Therapeutic receptor targets for lower urinary tract dysfunction. Naunyn Schmiedeberg's Arch Pharmacol. 2008;377:437–48.
7. Andersson K-E. Antimuscarinics for treatment of overactive bladder. Lancet Neurol. 2004;3:46–53.
8. Andersson K-E, Chapple CR, Cardozo L, Cruz F, Hashim H, Michel MC, et al. Pharmacological treatment of overactive bladder: report from the International Consultation on Incontinence. Curr Opin Urol. 2009;19:380–94.
9. Thiagamoorthy G, Cardozo L, Robinson D. Current and future pharmacotherapy for treating overactive bladder. Expert Opin Pharmacother. 2016;17:1317–25.
10. Mitchelson F. Muscarinic receptor agonists and antagonists: effects on ocular function. Handb Exp Pharmacol. 2012;263–98.
11. Ehlert FJ, Pak KJ, Griffin MT. Muscarinic agonists and antagonists: effects on gastrointestinal function. Handb Exp Pharmacol. 2012;343–74.
12. Yoshida M, Inadome A, Maeda Y, Satoji Y, Masunaga K, Sugiyama Y, et al. Non-neuronal cholinergic system in human bladder urothelium. Urology. 2006;67:425–30.
13. Gibson W, Johnson T, Kirschner-Hermanns R, Kuchel G, Markland A, Orme S, et al. Incontinence in frail elderly persons: report of the 6th International Consultation on Incontinence. Neurourol Urodyn. 2021;40:38–54.
14. Kraus SR, Bavendam T, Brake T, Griebling TL. Vulnerable elderly patients and overactive bladder syndrome. Drugs Aging. 2010;27:697–713.
15. Kraus SR, Ruiz-Cerdá JL, Martire D, Wang JT, Wagg AS. Efficacy and tolerability of fesoterodine in older and younger subjects with overactive bladder. Urology. 2010;76:1350–7.
16. Burgio KL, Goode PS, Johnson TM, Hammontree L, Ouslander JG, Markland AD, et al. Behavioral versus drug treatment for overactive bladder in men: the Male Overactive Bladder Treatment in Veterans (MOTIVE) Trial. J Am Geriatr Soc. 2011;59:2209–16.
17. Burgio KL, Kraus SR, Johnson TM, Markland AD, Vaughan CP, Li P, et al. Effectiveness of combined behavioral and drug therapy for overactive bladder symptoms in men: a randomized clinical trial. JAMA Intern Med. 2020;180:411–9.
18. Callegari E, Malhotra B, Bungay PJ, Webster R, Fenner KS, Kempshall S, et al. A comprehensive non-clinical evaluation of the CNS penetration potential of antimuscarinic agents for the treatment of overactive bladder. Br J Clin Pharmacol. 2011;72:235–46.
19. Jakobsen SM, Kersten H, Molden E. Evaluation of brain anticholinergic activities of urinary spasmolytic drugs using a high-throughput radio receptor bioassay. J Am Geriatr Soc. 2011;59:501–5.
20. Welk B, Richardson K, Panicker JN. The cognitive effect of anticholinergics for patients with overactive bladder. Nat Rev Urol. 2021;18:686–700.

21. Kay GG, Abou-Donia MB, Messer WS, Murphy DG, Tsao JW, Ouslander JG. Antimuscarinic drugs for overactive bladder and their potential effects on cognitive function in older patients. J Am Geriatr Soc. 2005;53:2195–201.
22. Chew ML, Mulsant BH, Pollock BG, Lehman ME, Greenspan A, Mahmoud RA, et al. Anticholinergic activity of 107 medications commonly used by older adults. J Am Geriatr Soc. 2008;56:1333–41.
23. Ancelin ML, Artero S, Portet F, Dupuy A-M, Touchon J, Ritchie K. Non-degenerative mild cognitive impairment in elderly people and use of anticholinergic drugs: longitudinal cohort study. BMJ. 2006;332:455–9.
24. Campbell N, Boustani M, Limbil T, Ott C, Fox C, Maidment I, et al. The cognitive impact of anticholinergics: a clinical review. Clin Interv Aging. 2009;4:225–33.
25. Fox C, Richardson K, Maidment ID, Savva GM, Matthews FE, Smithard D, et al. Anticholinergic medication use and cognitive impairment in the older population: the medical research council cognitive function and ageing study. J Am Geriatr Soc. 2011;59:1477–83.
26. Fader M, Glickman S, Haggar V, Barton R, Brooks R, Malone-Lee J. Intravesical atropine compared to oral oxybutynin for neurogenic detrusor overactivity: a double-blind, randomized crossover trial. J Urol. 2007;177:208–13; discussion 213.
27. Nicholas RS, Friede T, Hollis S, Young CA. WITHDRAWN: anticholinergics for urinary symptoms in multiple sclerosis. Cochrane Database Syst Rev. 2015;2015:CD004193.
28. Yamada S, Ito Y, Nishijima S, Kadekawa K, Sugaya K. Basic and clinical aspects of antimuscarinic agents used to treat overactive bladder. Pharmacol Ther. 2018;189:130–48.
29. McFerren SC, Gomelsky A. Treatment of overactive bladder in the elderly female: the case for trospium, oxybutynin, fesoterodine and darifenacin. Drugs Aging. 2015;32:809–19.
30. Araklitis G, Robinson D, Cardozo L. Cognitive effects of anticholinergic load in women with overactive bladder. Clin Interv Aging. 2020;15:1493–503.
31. Chapple CR, Van Kerrebroeck PE, Jünemann K-P, Wang JT, Brodsky M. Comparison of fesoterodine and tolterodine in patients with overactive bladder. BJU Int. 2008;102:1128–32.
32. Vasudeva P, Kumar A, Yadav S, Kumar N, Chaudhry N, Prasad V, et al. Neurological safety and efficacy of darifenacin and mirabegron for the treatment of overactive bladder in patients with history of cerebrovascular accident: a prospective study. Neurourol Urodyn. 2021;40:2041–7.
33. Van Meel TD, De Wachter S, Wyndaele JJ. The effect of intravesical oxybutynin on the ice water test and on electrical perception thresholds in patients with neurogenic detrusor overactivity. Neurourol Urodyn. 2010;29:391–4.
34. Novara G, Galfano A, Secco S, D'Elia C, Cavalleri S, Ficarra V, et al. A systematic review and meta-analysis of randomized controlled trials with antimuscarinic drugs for overactive bladder. Eur Urol. 2008;54:740–63.
35. Chapple CR, Khullar V, Gabriel Z, Muston D, Bitoun CE, Weinstein D. The effects of antimuscarinic treatments in overactive bladder: an update of a systematic review and meta-analysis. Eur Urol. 2008;54:543–62.
36. Huang W, Zong H, Zhou X, Wang T, Zhang Y. Efficacy and safety of propiverine hydrochloride for overactive bladder in adult: a systematic review and meta-analysis. Indian J Surg. 2015;77:1369–77.
37. McKeage K. Propiverine: a review of its use in the treatment of adults and children with overactive bladder associated with idiopathic or neurogenic detrusor overactivity, and in men with lower urinary tract symptoms. Clin Drug Investig. 2013;33:71–91.
38. Arcaniolo D, Conquy S, Tarcan T. Flavoxate: present and future. Eur Rev Med Pharmacol Sci. 2015;19:719–31.
39. Sweeney P, Mutambirwa S, Van An N, Sharma JB, Vanamail P. Flavoxate in the symptomatic treatment of overactive bladder: a meta-analysis. Eur Rev Med Pharmacol Sci. 2016;20:3703–12.
40. Velasco C, Guarneri L, Leonardi A, Testa R. Effects of intravenous and infravesical administration of suramin, terazosin and BMY 7378 on bladder instability in conscious rats with bladder outlet obstruction. BJU Int. 2003;92:131–6.

41. Tatemichi S, Akiyama K, Kobayashi M, Yamazaki Y, Yokoyama O, Uruno T. A selective alpha1A-adrenoceptor antagonist inhibits detrusor overactivity in a rat model of benign prostatic hyperplasia. J Urol. 2006;176:1236–41.
42. Nagase K, Ito H, Aoki Y, Tanase K, Akino H, Yokoyama O. Co-administration of an α(1)-blocker improves the efficacy and safety of antimuscarinic agents in rats with detrusor overactivity. Int J Urol. 2011;18:836–43.
43. Rechberger T, Wróbel A. Evaluating vibegron for the treatment of overactive bladder. Expert Opin Pharmacother. 2021;22:9–17.
44. Krauwinkel W, van Dijk J, Schaddelee M, Eltink C, Meijer J, Strabach G, et al. Pharmacokinetic properties of mirabegron, a β3-adrenoceptor agonist: results from two phase I, randomized, multiple-dose studies in healthy young and elderly men and women. Clin Ther. 2012;34:2144–60.
45. Giarenis I, Robinson D, Cardozo L. Overactive bladder and the β3-adrenoceptor agonists: current strategy and future prospects. Drugs. 2015;75:1707–13.
46. Chapple CR, Cardozo L, Nitti VW, Siddiqui E, Michel MC. Mirabegron in overactive bladder: a review of efficacy, safety, and tolerability. Neurourol Urodyn. 2014;33:17–30.
47. Matta R, Gomes T, Juurlink D, Jarvi K, Herschorn S, Nam RK. Receipt of overactive bladder drugs and incident dementia: a population-based case-control study. Eur Urol Focus. 2021;8(5):1433–40.
48. Staskin D, Frankel J, Varano S, Shortino D, Jankowich R, Mudd PN. International phase III, randomized, double-blind, placebo and active controlled study to evaluate the safety and efficacy of vibegron in patients with symptoms of overactive bladder: EMPOWUR. J Urol. 2020;204:316–24.
49. Yoshimura N, de Groat WC. Neural control of the lower urinary tract. Int J Urol. 1997;4:111–25.
50. Angelico P, Guarneri L, Velasco C, Cova R, Leonardi A, Clarke DE, et al. Effect of cyclooxygenase inhibitors on the micturition reflex in rats: correlation with inhibition of cyclooxygenase isozymes. BJU Int. 2006;97:837–46.
51. de Jongh R, van Koeveringe GA, van Kerrebroeck PEV, Markerink-van Ittersum M, de Vente J, Gillespie JI. The effects of exogenous prostaglandins and the identification of constitutive cyclooxygenase I and II immunoreactivity in the normal guinea pig bladder. BJU Int. 2007;100:419–29.
52. Stromberga Z, Chess-Williams R, Moro C. The five primary prostaglandins stimulate contractions and phasic activity of the urinary bladder urothelium, lamina propria and detrusor. BMC Urol. 2020;20:48.
53. Phelps C, Chess-Williams R, Moro C. The dependence of urinary bladder responses on extracellular calcium varies between muscarinic, histamine, 5-HT (serotonin), neurokinin, prostaglandin, and angiotensin receptor activation. Front Physiol. 2022;13:841181.
54. Montorsi F, Roehrborn C, Garcia-Penit J, Borre M, Roeleveld TA, Alimi J-C, et al. The effects of dutasteride or tamsulosin alone and in combination on storage and voiding symptoms in men with lower urinary tract symptoms (LUTS) and benign prostatic hyperplasia (BPH): 4-year data from the Combination of Avodart and Tamsulosin (CombAT) study. BJU Int. 2011;107:1426–31.
55. Haque N, Masumori N, Sakamoto S, Ye Z, Yoon S-J, Kuo H-C, et al. Superiority of dutasteride 0.5 mg and tamsulosin 0.2 mg for the treatment of moderate-to-severe benign prostatic hyperplasia in Asian men. Int J Urol. 2018;25:944–51.
56. Yamanishi T, Asakura H, Seki N, Tokunaga S. Efficacy and safety of combination therapy with tamsulosin, dutasteride and imidafenacin for the management of overactive bladder symptoms associated with benign prostatic hyperplasia: a multicenter, randomized, open-label, controlled trial (DIrecT study). Int J Urol. 2017;24:525–31.
57. Yamanishi T, Asakura H, Seki N, Tokunaga S. A 52-week multicenter randomized controlled study of the efficacy and safety of add-on dutasteride and imidafenacin to tamsulosin in patients with benign prostatic hyperplasia with remaining overactive bladder symptoms (DIrecT study). Low Urin Tract Symptoms. 2019;11:115–21.

58. Gratzke C, Bachmann A, Descazeaud A, Drake MJ, Madersbacher S, Mamoulakis C, et al. EAU guidelines on the assessment of non-neurogenic male lower urinary tract symptoms including benign prostatic obstruction. Eur Urol. 2015;67:1099–109.
59. Oelke M, Giuliano F, Mirone V, Xu L, Cox D, Viktrup L. Monotherapy with tadalafil or tamsulosin similarly improved lower urinary tract symptoms suggestive of benign prostatic hyperplasia in an international, randomised, parallel, placebo-controlled clinical trial. Eur Urol. 2012;61:917–25.
60. Andersson K-E, Uckert S, Stief C, Hedlund P. Phosphodiesterases (PDEs) and PDE inhibitors for treatment of LUTS. Neurourol Urodyn. 2007;26:928–33.
61. Andersson K-E. The use of pharmacotherapy for male patients with urgency and stress incontinence. Curr Opin Urol. 2014;24:571–7.
62. Urakami S, Ogawa K, Oka S, Hagiwara K, Nagamoto S, Anjiki H, et al. Effect of tadalafil add-on therapy in patients with persistant storage symptoms refractory to α1-adrenoceptor antagonist monotherapy for benign prostatic hyperplasia: a randomized pilot trial comparing tadalafil and solifenacin. Low Urin Tract Symptoms. 2019;11:109–14.
63. Yamanishi T, Kaga K, Sakata K, Yokoyama T, Kageyama S, Fuse M, et al. A randomized controlled study of the efficacy of tadalafil monotherapy versus combination of tadalafil and mirabegron for the treatment of persistent overactive bladder symptoms in men presenting with lower urinary tract symptoms (CONTACT study). Neurourol Urodyn. 2020;39:804–12.
64. Drake MJ. Emerging drugs for treatment of overactive bladder and detrusor overactivity. Expert Opin Emerg Drugs. 2008;13:431–46.
65. Pietra C, Poggesi E, Angelico P, Guarneri L, Testa R. Effects of some antidepressants on the volume-induced reflex contractions of the rat urinary bladder: lack of correlation with muscarinic receptors affinity. Pharmacol Res. 1990;22:421–32.
66. Han J, Jung JH, Bakker CJ, Ebell MH, Dahm P. Desmopressin for treating nocturia in men. Cochrane Database Syst Rev. 2017;10:CD012059.
67. Barakat B, Franke K, May M, Gauger U, Vögeli T-A. Efficacy and safety of desmopressin on frequency and urgency in female patients with overactive bladder and nocturia, current clinical features and outcomes: a systematic review. Asian J Urol. 2022;9:27–34.
68. Rovner ES, Raymond K, Andruczyk E, Juul KV. Low-dose desmopressin and tolterodine combination therapy for treating nocturia in women with overactive bladder: a double-blind, randomized, controlled study. Low Urin Tract Symptoms. 2018;10:221–30.
69. Friedman FM, Weiss JP. Desmopressin in the treatment of nocturia: clinical evidence and experience. Ther Adv Urol. 2013;5:310–7.
70. Yokoyama T, Nozaki K, Fujita O, Nose H, Inoue M, Kumon H. Role of C afferent fibers and monitoring of intravesical resiniferatoxin therapy for patients with idiopathic detrusor overactivity. J Urol. 2004;172:596–600.
71. He F, Ag L. Use of vanilloids in urologic disorders. Progress in drug research Fortschritte der Arzneimittelforschung Progres des recherches pharmaceutiques. Prog Drug Res. 2014;68:307–17. https://pubmed.ncbi.nlm.nih.gov/24941675/. [cited 2022 Nov 28].
72. MacDonald R, Fink HA, Huckabay C, Monga M, Wilt TJ. Botulinum toxin for treatment of urinary incontinence due to detrusor overactivity: a systematic review of effectiveness and adverse effects. Spinal Cord. 2007;45:535–41.
73. Chen J-L, Kuo H-C. Clinical application of intravesical botulinum toxin type A for overactive bladder and interstitial cystitis. Investig Clin Urol. 2020;61:S33–42.
74. Cruz F, Dinis P. Resiniferatoxin and botulinum toxin type A for treatment of lower urinary tract symptoms. Neurourol Urodyn. 2007;26:920–7.
75. Abrams P, Cardozo L, Fall M, Griffiths D, Rosier P, Ulmsten U, et al. The standardisation of terminology of lower urinary tract function: report from the Standardisation Sub-committee of the International Continence Society. Neurourol Urodyn. 2002;21:167–78.
76. Tsakiris P, de la Rosette JJ, Michel MC, Oelke M. Pharmacologic treatment of male stress urinary incontinence: systematic review of the literature and levels of evidence. Eur Urol. 2008;53:53 9.

77. Brune ME, O'Neill AB, Gauvin DM, Katwala SP, Altenbach RJ, Brioni JD, et al. Comparison of alpha 1-adrenoceptor agonists in canine urethral pressure profilometry and abdominal leak point pressure models. J Urol. 2001;166:1555–9.
78. Cornu J-N, Merlet B, Ciofu C, Mouly S, Peyrat L, Sèbe P, et al. Duloxetine for mild to moderate postprostatectomy incontinence: preliminary results of a randomised, placebo-controlled trial. Eur Urol. 2011;59:148–54.
79. Kotecha P, Sahai A, Malde S. Use of duloxetine for postprostatectomy stress urinary incontinence: a systematic review. Eur Urol Focus. 2021;7:618–28.
80. Okabe YT, Shimizu S, Suetake Y, Matsui-Hirai H, Hasegawa S, Takanari K, et al. Biological characterization of adipose-derived regenerative cells used for the treatment of stress urinary incontinence. Int J Urol. 2021;28:115–24.
81. Gotoh M, Shimizu S, Yamamoto T, Ishizuka O, Yamanishi T, Mizokami A, et al. Regenerative treatment for male stress urinary incontinence by periurethral injection of adipose-derived regenerative cells: outcome of the ADRESU study. Int J Urol. 2020;27:859–65.
82. Yamanishi T, Ishizuka O, Shimizu S, Kobayashi Y, Kinoshita F, Yamamoto T, et al. Influence of background characteristics in responders of regenerative therapy by periurethral injection of adipose-derived regenerative cells for male stress urinary incontinence. Low Urin Tract Symptoms. 2022;14:273–80.
83. Serlin DC, Heidelbaugh JJ, Stoffel JT. Urinary retention in adults: evaluation and initial management. Am Fam Physician. 2018;98:496–503.
84. Buckley BS, Lapitan MCM. Drugs for treatment of urinary retention after surgery in adults. Cochrane Database Syst Rev. 2010;CD008023.
85. Sirisreetreerux P, Wattanayingcharoenchai R, Rattanasiri S, Pattanaprateep O, Numthavaj P, Thakkinstian A. Medical and non-medical interventions for post-operative urinary retention prevention: network meta-analysis and risk-benefit analysis. Ther Adv Urol. 2021;13:17562872211022296.
86. Torres B, Serakides R, Caldeira F, Gomes M, Melo E. The ameliorating effect of dantrolene on the morphology of urinary bladder in spinal cord injured rats. Pathol Res Pract. 2011;207:775–9.
87. Te AE. A modern rationale for the use of phenoxybenzamine in urinary tract disorders and other conditions. Clin Ther. 2002;24:851–61; discussion 837.
88. Black CJ, Ford AC. Chronic idiopathic constipation in adults: epidemiology, pathophysiology, diagnosis and clinical management. Med J Aust. 2018;209:86–91.
89. Thompson WG, Longstreth GF, Drossman DA, Heaton KW, Irvine EJ, Müller-Lissner SA. Functional bowel disorders and functional abdominal pain. Gut. 1999;45 Suppl 2:II43–7.
90. Bharucha AE, Wald A, Enck P, Rao S. Functional anorectal disorders. Gastroenterology. 2006;130:1510–8.
91. Longstreth GF, Thompson WG, Chey WD, Houghton LA, Mearin F, Spiller RC. Functional bowel disorders. Gastroenterology. 2006;130:1480–91.
92. Sharma A, Rao S. Constipation: pathophysiology and current therapeutic approaches. Handb Exp Pharmacol. 2017;239:59–74.
93. Rao SSC. Dyssynergic defecation and biofeedback therapy. Gastroenterol Clin N Am. 2008;37:569–86. viii
94. Camilleri M. Gastrointestinal motility disorders in neurologic disease. J Clin Invest. 2021;131:e143771.
95. Li Y-W, Yu Y-J, Fei F, Zheng M-Y, Zhang S-W. High-resolution colonic manometry and its clinical application in patients with colonic dysmotility: a review. World J Clin Cases. 2019;7:2675–86.
96. Ge X, Zhao W, Ding C, Tian H, Xu L, Wang H, et al. Potential role of fecal microbiota from patients with slow transit constipation in the regulation of gastrointestinal motility. Sci Rep. 2017;7:441.
97. Chey WD, Kurlander J, Eswaran S. Irritable bowel syndrome: a clinical review. JAMA. 2015;313:949–58.
98. Halland M, Talley NJ. Fecal incontinence: mechanisms and management. Curr Opin Gastroenterol. 2012;28:57–62.

99. Varma MG, Brown JS, Creasman JM, Thom DH, Van Den Eeden SK, Beattie MS, et al. Fecal incontinence in females older than aged 40 years: who is at risk? Dis Colon Rectum. 2006;49:841–51.
100. Whitehead WE, Borrud L, Goode PS, Meikle S, Mueller ER, Tuteja A, et al. Fecal incontinence in US adults: epidemiology and risk factors. Gastroenterology. 2009;137:512–7, 517.e1–2.
101. Rey E, Choung RS, Schleck CD, Zinsmeister AR, Locke GR, Talley NJ. Onset and risk factors for fecal incontinence in a US community. Am J Gastroenterol. 2010;105:412–9.
102. Whitehead WE, Rao SSC, Lowry A, Nagle D, Varma M, Bitar KN, et al. Treatment of fecal incontinence: state of the science summary for the National Institute of Diabetes and Digestive and Kidney Diseases workshop. Am J Gastroenterol. 2015;110:138–46; quiz 147.
103. Read M, Read NW, Barber DC, Duthie HL. Effects of loperamide on anal sphincter function in patients complaining of chronic diarrhea with fecal incontinence and urgency. Dig Dis Sci. 1982;27:807–14.
104. Santoro GA, Eitan BZ, Pryde A, Bartolo DC. Open study of low-dose amitriptyline in the treatment of patients with idiopathic fecal incontinence. Dis Colon Rectum. 2000;43:1676–81; discussion 1681–1682.
105. Bharucha AE, Seide BM, Zinsmeister AR. The effects of clonidine on symptoms and anorectal sensorimotor function in women with faecal incontinence. Aliment Pharmacol Ther. 2010;32:681–8.
106. Norton C, Cody JD, Hosker G. Biofeedback and/or sphincter exercises for the treatment of faecal incontinence in adults. Cochrane Database Syst Rev. 2006;CD002111.
107. Adriani A, Ribaldone DG, Astegiano M, Durazzo M, Saracco GM, Pellicano R. Irritable bowel syndrome: the clinical approach. Panminerva Med. 2018;60:213–22.
108. Lovell RM, Ford AC. Global prevalence of and risk factors for irritable bowel syndrome: a meta-analysis. Clin Gastroenterol Hepatol. 2012;10:712–721.e4.
109. Saha L. Irritable bowel syndrome: pathogenesis, diagnosis, treatment, and evidence-based medicine. World J Gastroenterol. 2014;20:6759–73.
110. Bonetto S, Fagoonee S, Battaglia E, Grassini M, Saracco GM, Pellicano R. Recent advances in the treatment of irritable bowel syndrome. Pol Arch Intern Med. 2021;131:709–15.
111. Goldstein I, Lue TF, Padma-Nathan H, et al. Oral sildenafil in the treatment of erectile dysfunction. N Engl J Med. 1998;338(20):1397–404.
112. Blok BF, Holstege G. The central nervous system control of micturition in cats and humans. Behav Brain Res. 1998;92:119–25.
113. Blok BF, Willemsen AT, Holstege G. A PET study on brain control of micturition in humans. Brain. 1997;120(Pt 1):111–21.
114. Sugaya K, Nishijima S, Miyazato M, Ogawa Y. Central nervous control of micturition and urine storage. J Smooth Muscle Res. 2005;41:117–32.
115. Scaglione F, Donde S, Hassan TA, et al. Phosphodiesterase type 5 inhibitors for the treatment of erectile dysfunction: pharmacology and clinical impact of the sildenafil citrate orodispersible tablet formulation. Clin Ther. 2017;39(2):370–7.
116. Hatzimouratidis K, et al. Pharmacotherapy for erectile dysfunction: recommendations from the fourth International Consultation for Sexual Medicine (ICSM 2015). J Sex Med. 2016;13(4):465–88.
117. Seftel AD. Phosphodiesterase type 5 inhibitor differentiation based on selectivity, pharmacokinetic, and efficacy profiles. Clin Cardiol. 2004;27(S1):14–9.
118. Porst H, et al. SOP conservative (medical and mechanical) treatment of erectile dysfunction. J Sex Med. 2013;10(1):130–71.
119. Ferguson JE, Carson CC. Phosphodiesterase type 5 inhibitors as a treatment for erectile dysfunction: current information and new horizons. Arab J Urol. 2013;11(3):222–9.
120. McCullough AR. Four-year review of sildenafil citrate. Rev Urol. 2002;4 Suppl 3:S26–38.
121. Goldstein I, Tseng LJ, Creanga D, et al. Efficacy and safety of sildenafil by age in men with erectile dysfunction. J Sex Med. 2016;13(5):852–9.

122. Jannini EA, Isidori AM, Gravina GL, et al. The ENDOTRIAL study: a spontaneous, open-label, randomized, multicenter, crossover study on the efficacy of sildenafil, tadalafil, and vardenafil in the treatment of erectile dysfunction. J Sex Med. 2009;6(9):2547–60.
123. Corona G, Rastrelli G, Burri A, et al. The safety and efficacy of Avanafil, a new 2nd generation PDE5i: comprehensive review and meta-analysis. Expert Opin Drug Saf. 2016;15(2):237–47.
124. Damle B, Duczynski G, Jeffers BW, et al. Pharmacokinetics of a novel oro-dispersible tablet of sildenafil in healthy subjects. Clin Ther. 2014;36(2):236–44.
125. Radicioni M, Castiglioni C, Giori A, et al. Bioequivalence study of a new sildenafil 100 mg orodispersible film compared to the conventional filmcoated 100 mg tablet administered to healthy male volunteers. Drug Des Devel Ther. 2017;11:1183–92.
126. Gittelman M, McMahon CG, Rodríguez-Rivera JA, et al. The POTENT II randomised trial: efficacy and safety of an orodispersible vardenafil formulation for the treatment of erectile dysfunction. Int J Clin Pract. 2010;64(5):594–603.
127. Liao X, Qiu S, Bao Y, et al. Comparative efficacy and safety of phosphodiesterase type 5 inhibitors for erectile dysfunction in diabetic men: a Bayesian network meta-analysis of randomized controlled trials. World J Urol. 2019;37(6):1061–74.
128. Berner MM, Kriston L, Harms A. Efficacy of PDE-5-inhibitors for erectile dysfunction. A comparative meta-analysis of fixed-dose regimen randomized controlled trials administering the International Index of Erectile Function in broad-spectrum populations. Int J Imp Res. 2006;18(3):229–35.
129. Belew D, Klaassen Z, Lewis RW. Intracavernosal injection for the diagnosis, evaluation, and treatment of erectile dysfunction: a review. Sex Med Rev. 2015;3(1):11–23.
130. Duncan C, Omran GJ, Teh J, et al. Erectile dysfunction: a global review of intracavernosal injectables. World J Urol. 2019;37(6):1007–14.
131. Chung E. A review of current and emerging therapeutic options for erectile dysfunction. Med Sci. 2019;7(9):91–7.
132. Hanchanale V, Eardley I. Alprostadil for the treatment of impotence. Expert Opin Pharmacother. 2014;15(3):421–8.
133. Lea AP, Bryson HM, Balfour JA. Intracavernous alprostadil: a review of its pharmacodynamic and pharmacokinetic properties and therapeutic potential in erectile dysfunction. Drugs Aging. 1996;8(1):56–74.
134. Porst H. The rationale for prostaglandin E1 in erectile failure: a survey of worldwide experience. J Urol. 1996;155(3):802–15.
135. Porst H, Buvat J, Meuleman E, et al. Intracavernous alprostadil alfadex—an effective and well tolerated treatment for erectile dysfunction. Results of a long-term European study. Int J Impot Res. 1998;10(4):225–31.
136. Costa P, Potempa AJ. Intraurethral alprostadil for erectile dysfunction: a review of the literature. Drugs. 2012;72(17):2243–54.
137. Hatzimouratidis IK, Giuliano F, Moncada, et al. EAU guidelines on erectile dysfunction, premature ejaculation, penile curvature and priapism. 2016.
138. Cai T, Palumbo F, Liguori G, et al. The intra-meatal application of alprostadil cream (Vitaros®) improves drug efficacy and patient's satisfaction: results from a randomized, two-administration route, crossover clinical trial. Int J Impot Res. 2019;31(2):119–2.

7 Coloproctological Complications After Radical Prostatectomy

Veronica De Simone and Carlo Ratto

Since the implementation of prostate-specific antigen (PSA) testing, there has been a significant change toward more favorable stages in newly identified cases of prostate cancer (PCa), resulting in roughly 81% of cases being identified as clinically localized. At present, the recommended approaches for managing clinically localized PCa are founded on solid evidence and encompass options such as active surveillance (AS), surgical intervention, external beam radiotherapy (EBRT), and brachytherapy (BT) [1].

Historical datasets involving patients treated with RP showcased substantial complication rates, ranging from one-third to one-half of cases. These complications encompassed rectal injuries, bladder neck contractures, bleeding, ureteral damage, fistulas connecting the bladder or rectum, venous blood clot formation, and persistent urinary incontinence [2, 3]. In fact, the adverse events after such surgery negatively impact disease-specific QoL of the affected patients. Luckily, owing to advancements in research, only a minority of individuals with initial-stage PCa progresses into metastatic conditions and faces cancer-related mortality within a span of 10–15 years. Nonetheless, this highlights the importance of comprehending the enduring consequences of treatments on the quality of life specific to the disease. Furthermore, performing RP after prior radiotherapy introduces greater technical

V. De Simone (✉)
Proctology and Pelvic Foor Surgery Unit, Fatebenefratelli Isola Tiberina – Gemelli Isola, Rome, Italy

C. Ratto
Proctology and Pelvic Foor Surgery Unit, Fatebenefratelli Isola Tiberina – Gemelli Isola, Rome, Italy

Department of Medical and Surgical Sciences, Università Cattolica del Sacro Cuore, Rome, Italy

G. Lamberti, C. De Nunzio (eds.), *Bladder, Bowel and Sexual Dysfunctions Rehabilitation after Radical Prostatectomy*, Urodynamics, Neurourology and Pelvic Floor Dysfunctions, https://doi.org/10.1007/978-3-031-76341-0_7

complexity and heightened risk of notable complications compared to cases without prior radiotherapy.

Bowel complication after RP can occur with or without prior radiotherapy, and they include alterations in bowel habits, such as postoperative ileus or increased frequency of bowel movements, urgency, or diarrhea, and recto-anal problems including rectal bleeding, irritation, and discomfort [4]. Innervation and anatomy of the anal canal may be injured by perineal RP leading to fecal incontinence, intended as unintentional leakage of stool resulting in difficulty in controlling bowel movements with a huge impact on a person's QoL. However, studies in literature demonstrated that the prevalence of anal incontinence in the elderly population is approximately 6–11%, and the most important risk factor for this disorder is age. Indeed, a significant decrease in the sphincter symmetry index after perineal prostatectomy has been reported, but except for the sphincter asymmetry index, perineal prostatectomy does not show to affect anal continence parameters [5, 6].

Fecal incontinence after RP has always been underestimated. Bishoff et al. conducted a study revealing that fecal incontinence rates were 5% among those who had retropubic RP, according to a telephone survey. Additionally, they found that 50% of surveyed patients had not disclosed their problem to their physicians. Subsequently, they conducted a follow-up mail survey to support this discovery [7, 8].

Another possible complication rarely reported in literature concerns scarring or narrowing of the rectum (rectal stricture or stenosis) which can lead to difficulties with bowel movements, including constipation or incomplete evacuation. Moreover, pelvic floor muscles play a crucial role in controlling bowel movements. Surgery can sometimes disrupt these muscles, leading to pelvic floor dysfunction. This may result in difficulties with bowel control and may require physical therapy or other treatments to improve muscle function. However, usually radiotherapy patients experience more bowel dysfunction than do RP patients. About half as many RP patients as radiotherapy patients report diarrhea, bowel urgency, or painful hemorrhoids. However, Potoskyn et al. reported in their study that around 20% of patients who underwent RP experienced recurrent diarrhea, while 16% reported bowel urgency symptoms, and 9.5% painful hemorrhoids. The percentage of patients reporting painful bowel movements was reported to be nearly the same in both treatment groups and it was around 10.7%. Furthermore, around 5% of both RP- and external beam radiotherapy (EBRT)-treated patients suffered from frequent, painful, or urgent bowel movements [9]. Another systematic review regarding QoL after treatment for PCa reported that the surgical approach as RP exhibited adverse implications especially for maintaining urinary continence and sexual function; in contrast, EBRT was more linked to a reduction in bowel function, which was particularly pronounced during the initial year posttreatment. However, others report that surgery resulted in more incontinence but less irritating/obstructive symptoms than EBRT [1]. In terms of bowel function, Nossiter et al. reported no difference comparing robot-assisted radical prostatectomy (RARP), laparoscopic radical prostatectomy (LRP), or open retropubic radical prostatectomy (ORP) approaches [10].

Management of bowel complications after RP involves a multifaceted approach aimed at identifying and addressing the specific issues affecting the bowel. As mentioned, while bowel complications are relatively uncommon after this surgery, they can be serious. Management encompasses early recognition of signs and symptoms, a specific diagnostic evaluation through tests such as imaging studies (e.g., CT scan, MRI, or ultrasound), endoscopy (colonoscopy, sigmoidoscopy), and laboratory tests, as well as consultation with specialists such as gastroenterologists or colorectal surgeons. Treatment options vary between conservative management in the case of mild or early-onset complications, including pain control and medication (e.g., antispasmodics for bowel spasms), and close monitoring of symptoms, and surgical intervention, which is dedicated to addressing organic disorders such as bowel injury, perforations, and fistulas.

The incidence of rectal injury after RP ranges between 0.12% and 9% and have decreased of 26% from years 2003–2006 to 2009–2012, with most of the studies reporting rates less than 0.5% [3]; the same happened concerning rectovesical fistula rate, today estimated to be <1% which however, even though rare, is another dreaded and associated complication [11].

Although an intraoperative rectal injury stands out as the primary risk contributor to rectourethral fistula (RUF) (Fig. 7. 1) [12], there exist other inherent factors

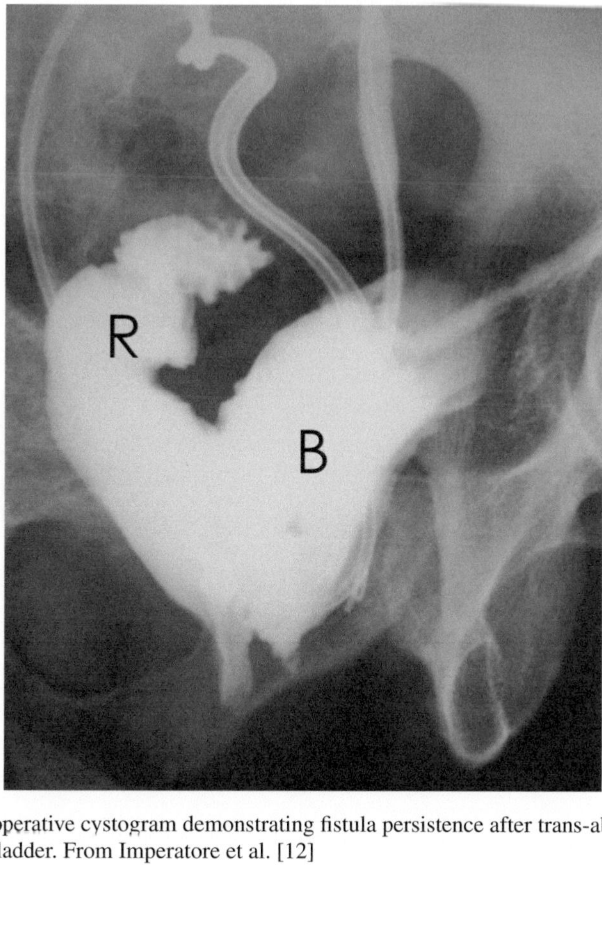

Fig. 7.1 Post-operative cystogram demonstrating fistula persistence after trans-abdominal repair. R: rectum, B: bladder. From Imperatore et al. [12]

inevitably linked to this complication. Notable among these factors are extracapsular disease presence, higher Gleason scores indicating more advanced cancer, broader surgical excisions, as well as previous exposure to radiotherapy or hormone therapy. The clinical manifestation of an RUF encompasses a combination of distinctive clinical markers including pneumaturia (passage of air in urine), fecaluria (presence of feces in urine), anal urinary discharge, intractable diarrhea, and recurrent infections within the urinary tract [3, 13, 14]. A provisional approach involving conservative management, which combines a low-residue diet with temporary urinary and/or fecal diversion, exhibits a range of effectiveness (with success rates spanning from 14% to 100%). This strategy has the potential to induce spontaneous closure within a 3-month timeframe, particularly in cases involving straightforward fistulas. However, patients displaying symptoms like fecaluria or pneumaturia necessitate immediate intervention, which often involves creating a diverting colostomy. This proactive measure is essential to avert the risk of recurring and potentially severe urinary infections, albeit in a smaller subset of cases. When this option has failed, a primary closure of the fistula (via transabdominal, transperineal, or transsphincteric approach), a flap, or a graft interposition from the buccal mucosa can be attempted (Figs. 7. 2 and 7. 3) [1, 11–13].

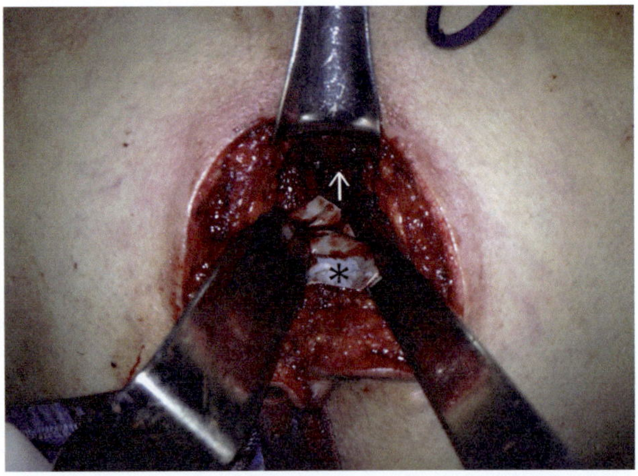

Fig. 7.2 The porcine dermal graft is positioned to cover the defect. Asterisk: graft, arrow: UVA. From Imperatore et al. [12]

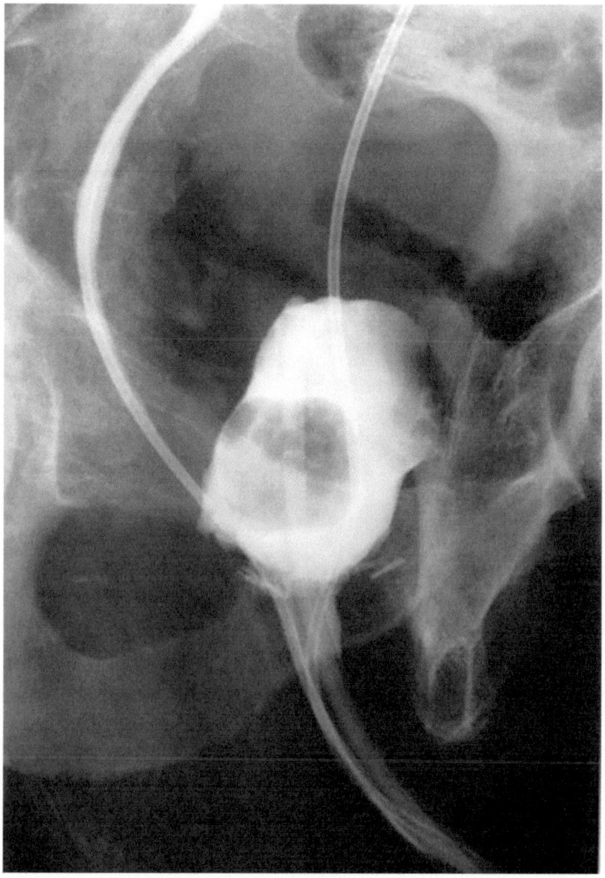

Fig. 7.3 Post-operative cystogram demonstrating fistula healing after transperineal repair. From Imperatore et al. [12]

References

1. Lardas M, Liew M, van den Bergh RC, De Santis M, Bellmunt J, Van den Broeck T, et al. Quality of life outcomes after primary treatment for clinically localised prostate cancer: a systematic review. Eur Urol. 2017;72:869–85.
2. Sacco E, Prayer-Galetti T, Pinto F, Fracalanza S, Betto G, Pagano F, Artibani W. Urinary incontinence after radical prostatectomy: incidence by definition, risk factors and temporal trend in a large series with a long-term follow-up. BJU Int. 2006;97(6):1234–41.
3. Romito I, Giannarini G, Rossanese M, Mucciardi G, Simonato A, Ficarra V. Incidence of rectal injury after radical prostatectomy: a systematic review and meta-analysis. Eur Urol Open Sci. 2023;52:85–99.
4. Park JS, Kim J, Jang WS, Heo JE, Elghiaty A, Rha KH, et al. Management of postoperative ileus after robot-assisted laparoscopic prostatectomy. Medicine (United States). 2018;97(44):e13036.
5. Kirschner-Hermanns R, Borchers H, Reineke T, Willis S, Jakse G. Fecal incontinence after radical perineal prostatectomy: a prospective study. Urology. 2005;65(2):337–42.

6. Guilger NR, Jorge JMN, Costa RP, Salla FC, Teixeira MG, Nahas SC, et al. Influence of perineal prostatectomy on anal continence. Clinics. 2011;66(12):2007–12.
7. Korman HJ, Mulholland TL, Huang R. Preservation of fecal continence and bowel function after radical perineal and retropubic prostatectomy: a questionnaire-based outcomes study. Prostate Cancer Prostatic Dis. 2004;7(3):249–52.
8. Bishoff JT, et al. Incidence of fecal and urinary incontinence following radical perineal and retropubic prostatectomy in a national population. J Urol. 1998;160(2):454–8.
9. Potosky AL, Legler J, Albertsen PC, Stanford JL, Gilliland FD, Hamilton AS, et al. Health outcomes after prostatectomy or radiotherapy for prostate cancer: results from the prostate cancer outcomes study. J Natl Cancer Inst. 2000;92(19):1582–92. https://academic.oup.com/jnci/article/92/19/1582/2905955.
10. Nossiter J, Sujenthiran A, Charman SC, Cathcart PJ, Aggarwal A, Payne H, et al. Robot-assisted radical prostatectomy vs laparoscopic and open retropubic radical prostatectomy: functional outcomes 18 months after diagnosis from a national cohort study in England. Br J Cancer. 2018;118(4):489–94.
11. Amato A, Pellino G, Secondo P, Selvaggi F. Intersphincteric approach for rectourethral fistulas following radical prostatectomy. Tech Coloproctol. 2015;19(11):699–703.
12. Imperatore V, Creta M, Di Meo S, Buonopane R, Fusco F, Imbimbo C, Longo N, Mirone V. Transperineal repair of a persistent rectourethral fistula using a porcine dermal graft. Int J Surg Case Rep. 2014;5(11):800-2. https://doi.org/10.1016/j.ijscr.2014.09.019. Epub 2014 Sep 28. PMID: 25305599; PMCID: PMC4245663.
13. Ghandour R, Vaillant JC, Genser L. Recto-urethral fistula after radical prostatectomy. J Gastrointest Surg. 2022;26:2618–9.
14. Kurtz LE, Sheikh JM, Greenberg RE. Acute diarrhea caused by a rectovesical fistula after laparoscopic prostatectomy. Clin Gastroenterol Hepatol. 2010;8(6):A30.

Pelvic Floor Muscle Training and Biofeedback for Urinary, Bowel, and Erectile Dysfunction

8

Luisa De Palma, Elena Bertolucci, and Donatella Giraudo

8.1 Pelvic Floor Muscle Training

Pelvic floor muscle training (PFMT) is one of the recommended techniques for the prevention, treatment, and rehabilitation of radical prostatectomy-related complications. PFMT is considered as the first-line conservative treatment for urinary incontinence (UI), as suggested by the International Continence Society (ICS), and it has been proven to guarantee results for UI. Guided PFMT also improves adherence positively, promotes self-efficacy behavior among the participants, and helps in the closure of the urethral sphincter muscles, thus resulting in improvement in incontinence. Hence, it is prescribed for increasing strength, endurance, and muscle coordination. Although it is a treatment considered universally effective, there is a lack of standardized treatment protocols, regarding both preoperative and postoperative PFMT and its benefits: Data in the literature are scarce, and some results are controversial in the context of UI, bowel dysfunction, and erectile dysfunction (ED). Also, timing is not clear: The literature [1] takes into account effects of PFMT at 3, 6, and 12 months and it is not clear when to start, before and/or after surgical approach, and what is meant by late rehabilitation: beyond 6 months but within 12 or beyond 12 months? As indicated in literature [2], when rehabilitation started before surgery [3–7], the results were mixed in terms of efficacy on urinary incontinence.

L. De Palma
Physical, Rehabilitation Medicine and Spinal Cord Unit, Polyclinic of Bari, Bari, Italy

E. Bertolucci (✉)
Physical, rehabilitation Medicine and Spinal Cord Unit,
University Hospital Città della Salute e della Scienza, Torino, Italy

D. Giraudo
Urology Department, San Raffaele Hosp. Ville Turro, Milan, Italy

G. Lamberti, C. De Nunzio (eds.), *Bladder, Bowel and Sexual Dysfunctions Rehabilitation after Radical Prostatectomy*, Urodynamics, Neurourology and Pelvic Floor Dysfunctions, https://doi.org/10.1007/978-3-031-76341-0_8

After surgery, intensive and prolonged early PFMT may further increase the number of continent patients, and this improvement continues in the first 12 months. The second 6 months after surgery are still beneficial for recovery [7].

8.1.1 Pelvic Floor Muscle Training for Urinary Dysfunction

Urinary continence in men depends on the contributions from smooth muscle of the urethra and urethral constriction generated by contraction of three striated muscles: the striated urethral sphincter (SUS), puborectalis (PR), and bulbocavernosus (BC).

These striated muscles are active during urine storage, and their activation is greater with elevated intra-abdominal pressure such as coughing [8].

The treatment of prostate cancer depends on tumor stage and patient age. Radical prostatectomy, the treatment of choice, may be performed classically as open surgery or as laparoscopic or robotic-assisted laparoscopic surgery [9].

Radical prostatectomy inherently removes the entire prostate gland (in the section between the external sphincter or its innervation and the bladder neck), the prostatic segment of the urethra, and its smooth muscle (the internal sphincter), together with both seminal vesicles and bilateral pelvic lymph nodes. Surgery may also affect the bladder contractility and compliance, contributing to overactivity of the detrusor muscle.

The most common complications of surgical and radiotherapeutic treatments include urinary incontinence and erectile dysfunction. Fecal incontinence is less frequent, and it can occur especially in patients undergoing radiotherapy.

Post-prostatectomy incontinence (PPI) reduces postoperative quality of life. The majority of patients experience urinary incontinence immediately after RP, and in some cases, this incontinence is protracted.

Pelvic floor muscle training (PFMT), with or without biofeedback, promotes muscle contraction and accelerates recovery from PPI empowering function of striated urinary sphincter (SUS) and other striated muscles to compensate for the decrease in smooth muscle strength.

The rehabilitation treatment of the pelvic floor, often used as the first therapeutic approach in the management of urogenital dysfunctions, includes the treatment of alterations that affect not only the pelvic floor but also elements of the urological system, defecatory, genitosexual, postural, and pelvic statics. In order to identify the objectives of the therapy, before starting a pelvic floor rehabilitation program, it is essential to evaluate the integrity of the muscles and their contractility. However, digital rectal examination provides information on anal sphincter and puborectalis (PR) contraction but cannot provide information on the SUS and bulbocavernosus (BC), possible instead by transperineal ultrasound imaging, a noninvasive and validated method to evaluate and provide feedback of PR, SUS, and BC simultaneously [10].

The effects of the rehabilitation treatment are not yet fully understood. Normally, the individual should be able to contract and relax the pelvic floor both quickly and slowly on demand. If muscle function is impaired, voluntary contraction may not be visible and may be reduced or absent on intra-anal palpation.

The mechanism of action according to which this type of intervention should have had positive effects is based on the assumption that a strong and valid contraction closed the urethra by increasing the urethral pressure, so as to prevent the involuntary loss of urine following an increase in intra-abdominal pressure. Ultimately, muscle contraction would lead to the appearance of a reflex contraction which produces an increase in bladder pressure and inhibits detrusor overactivity.

The rehabilitation treatment must be adapted to the single individual and varies depending on the path for the duration and extent of the movement, for the position of the body and coordination depending on the respiratory acts. The evolution of rehabilitation techniques and scientific research have made it possible to abandon the idea of pelvic floor muscle training as a simple sequence of contraction and relaxation exercises and to direct the clinician toward a more structured and reasoned approach.

8.1.1.1 Presurgical Treatment

The various studies on management in the preoperative period are diversified in times and methods of implementation: only verbal instructions, PFMT, and PFMT + BFB. The ICI recommendations are difficult to interpret. The AUA underlines how the preoperative PFME/PFMT has not demonstrated its effectiveness, but since it is a risk-free therapy, pelvic floor exercises started 3–4 weeks before surgery can be offered to patients awaiting prostatectomy (grade C). On the contrary, the EAU guidelines underline with a grade 1b evidence that the preoperative PFMT does not add additional benefits to men awaiting prostatectomy, but in the recommendations, it is then limited to expressing a generic "offer instructions to men undergoing prostatectomy" (strong recommendation in 2020, reduced to weak and referred to PFMT with or without BFB/ES in 2022), without specifying the timing of pre- or postoperative.

Two reviews (Wu 2018 and Hall 2020) come to different conclusions: Wu [7] reports that the "supervised" PFMT results in percentages of continents higher than controls at 1, 3, 6, and even 12 months after the PR, but the addition of preoperative exercises would not provide superior results even 1 and 3 months after the PR. Hall [8], as also taken up in Mungovan's review of 2021 [9], concludes for better results in the training started in the preoperative period, without however differentiating the timing to which these results refer after RP.

8.1.1.2 Late Rehabilitation Treatment

The literature considers effects of PFME/PFMT at 3, 6, and 12 months, and it is not clear what is meant by late rehabilitation: more than 6 months but within 12 or more than 12 months? Few works on long-term treatment are as follows: Yokoyama et al. [10] but only on the administration of EXMI (extracorporeal magnetic innervation) 1 year after surgery and Goode et al. [11] on men with incontinence still present 1–17 years after intervention with the administration of behavioral therapy and BFB and ES, the addition of which did not produce additional efficacy.

Although nonsurgical options, such as pelvic floor muscle exercises (PFME), can speed continence recovery, patients who remain incontinent 1 year after the procedure or who have severe incontinence at 6 months may choose to undergo a surgical treatment (e.g., urinary sphincter) [12].

Evaluating the Timing for the Administration of PFME or PFMT:

- Before surgery, there were discordant results regarding efficacy on urinary incontinence.
- PFME or early intensive and prolonged PFMT may further increase the number of continent patients, and this improvement continues into the first 12 months. The second 6 months after surgery are still useful for healing.

In the context of treatment, the conscious involvement of patients is fundamental. The first phase is that of motor learning. It begins with the awareness of the pelvic anatomy and can take place through the use of anatomical tables or drawings, in a private and comfortable environment. Subsequently, the operator observes the perineal area and palpates the perineum, stretching the perineal area facilitating perception and muscle contraction.

The therapist can then encourage an awareness of the more anterior perineum by stretching the ischium cavernosum muscle and inviting the patient to contract the pelvic floor muscles, thus making it easier to feel the muscular engagement at the base of the penis.

Several training protocols have been proposed. Contractions may be accompanied by tactile feedback from the therapist, with two fingers resting under the scrotum (on the CFNP) to assess engagement tone and two fingers resting on the bulbocavernosus to produce a kind of stretch that facilitates engagement (stretch reflex or pre-penile maneuver) (Fig. 8.1) [13].

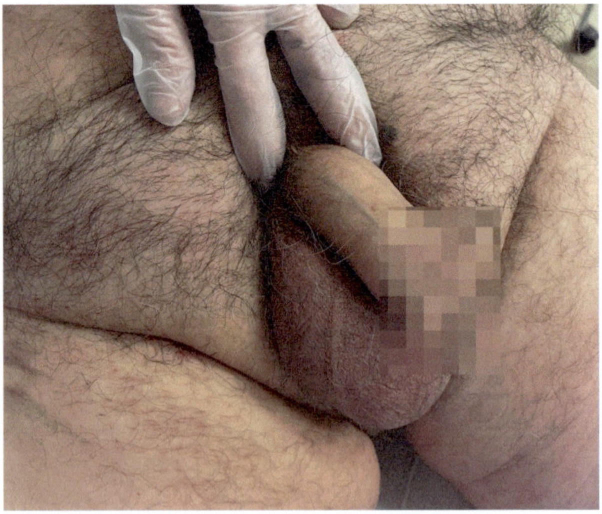

Fig. 8.1 Stretch reflex or pre-penile maneuver to facilitate voluntary contraction of the bulbocavernosus muscle

Once adequate phasicity and tonicity have been achieved (assessed by perineal testing), we can introduce a counter resistance to further increase voluntary engagement. Then using the endoanal maneuver (therapist's middle finger resting from the inside on the central fibrous nucleus of the perineum), the therapist can introduce a counter resistance directly on the muscle, using an outward stretching of the center of the perineum followed by the request to tighten the muscle, which will result in the introflexion of the muscle itself.

Once the individual movements and their sequence have been learned and perfected, the last phase of automation begins: The patient uses what he has learned and transfers the concepts learned into the various situations of daily life. During this phase, it is possible to reduce the therapy sessions and cyclically review the patient to check the correct execution of the movement and correct any errors. There are not enough studies to allow us to say the efficacy of PFMT. In addition, published evidence regarding the efficacy of existing PFMT programs for preventing and treating PPI is inconsistent.

The additional problem about rehabilitation concerns the PFMT regimens that vary considerably across the published studies. There are significant differences between each PFMT regimen regarding PFMT position (supine, sitting, or standing), contraction number, and duration or PFMT session frequency per day. Some authors [14] instructed the patients to perform a series of 10 contractions lasting 5 s with 10 s of muscular relaxation 3 times a day. Others propose a series of 15 contractions, and others propose 10 contractions lasting 10 s. Some other authors [2, 15] divide patients into a training of slow-twitch fibers and a training of fast-twitch fibers or instructed their patients to perform additional 3–4 fast contractions following each PFMT session (10 contractions of 6–8 s).

S, there is a need for further research to standardize procedures and determine the exact method for pelvic floor muscle exercise in men after radical prostatectomy.

8.1.2 Pelvic Floor Muscle Training for Bowel Dysfunction

The percentage of men reporting fecal incontinence and loose stools following radical prostatectomy is highly variable: It seems that the incidence rate from 4% to 15% is such only in prostatectomy with retropubic approach, while incidence is higher for radical perineal prostatectomy patients [16]. However, radical perineal prostatectomy patients have a significantly lower incidence of urinary incontinence than those treated with retropubic prostatectomy. Rates increases if prostate cancer is treated with radiotherapy. Bowel symptoms after radical prostatectomy might also be related to nerve-sparing or non-nerve-sparing surgery [17]. Nishikawa et al. [18] looked at bowel function during the first period after nerve-sparing or non-nerve-sparing radical prostatectomy that was significantly impaired but influenced by the degree of nerve-sparing surgery. Bowel function, however, is less impaired and less troublesome for men after prostatectomy. Bowel dysfunction symptoms are transient and normal bowel function is quickly recovered. The risk factors for developing fecal incontinence include advancing age, diarrhea, urinary incontinence, diabetes, hormone therapy, and previous rectal resection. The percentage may vary according to the severity of the disease before treatment, the extent of the resection, and the dose of pelvic radiotherapy. There are no randomized studies in the literature that provide for isolated use of PFMT without biofeedback for treatment of fecal incontinence post radical prostatectomy. It is possible that PFMT treatment could improve fecal incontinence, as well as urinary incontinence, but there are no specific protocols. They could still be prescribed in consideration of the fact that they do not present risks associated with the procedure and have a low cost.

8.1.3 Pelvic Floor Muscle Training for Erectile Dysfunction

Erectile dysfunction (ED) has been shown to affect 26–100% of men after RP. The period required for recovery of erectile function after surgery could vary from 6 to 48 months. However, 5 years after radical prostatectomy, only a third of patients reported having an erection firm enough for penetration.

ED is the main complication alongside urinary incontinence and affects heavily quality of life. Difficulties in achieving orgasm, deformity or shortening of the penis, altered fertility, and decreased sexual desire are associated.

For this reason, following radical prostatectomy, patients not only experience distressing physical side effects but also report significantly lower sexual confidence and sexual intimacy with their partners, anxiety relating to sexual penetration, depression, and a diminished sense of masculinity and self-confidence regarding their sexual abilities, especially if ED is associated with climacturia (loss of urine with orgasm).

These physical and psychological changes have led many physicians to develop programs to treat ED post RP. In addition to pharmacological therapy, vacuum erection devices and PFMT can be proposed, even if a high percentage of patients who starts treatment abandon it early because of loss of interest in sex, insufficient erection, and urethral pain and burning.

Erectile dysfunction following radical prostatectomy is caused by injury or removal of the cavernous nerves. It follows a reduction of nitric oxide required for mediating smooth muscle relaxation and vasodilation in normal penile erection. To overcome this problem, nerve-sparing techniques are increasingly widespread, and medication, vacuum compression pumps, and intracavernosal injections are now considered best practice to minimize side effects. However, these techniques are often prematurely abandoned because they are considered invasive by the patient, so patient compliance to treatment is poor.

Many different treatment strategies have been devised to improve ED in post-RP patients. Although there is little consensus with regard to the best strategy, treatment is undoubtedly better than leaving the tissue unassisted. PFMT is considered a non-invasive treatment for treating ED. It represents a conservative, well-tolerated, and low-cost treatment, providing for normal progression of erectile tissue recovery following RP even if it does not lead to a sudden improvement in sexual function.

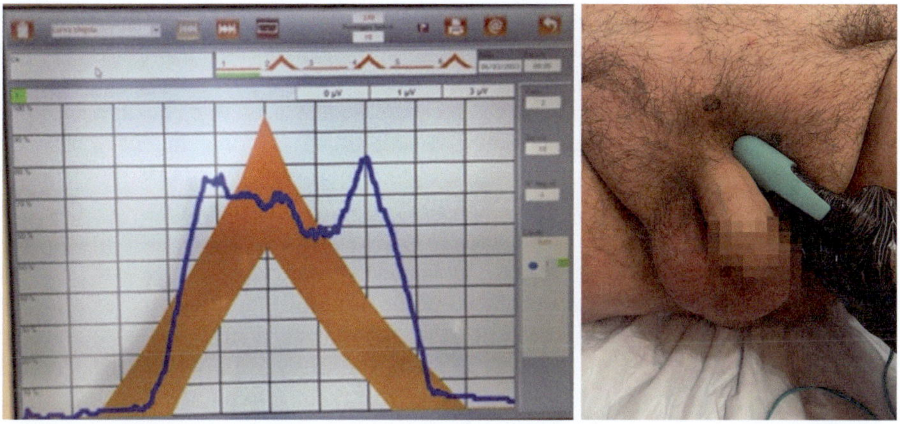

Fig. 8.2 BFB-EMG (electromyographic biofeedback) whit surface electrode to control the phasic contraction of the ischiocavernosus muscle

There have been no published studies regarding the potential impact of preoperative PFMT on subsequent ED, as well as for incontinence. When proposed, it usually consists with an intervention of greater exercise intensity and volume, both beginning approximately 5 weeks prior to RP and continuing for 3 months thereafter.

In erectile dysfunction (ED), the vascular reflex mechanism is not able to pump blood with enough pressure toward the cavernous body of the penis, and consequently, the penis erection cannot be maintained. The rigidity phase of the erection is insured by the correct function of the ischiocavernosus muscle, weakened by the use of the bladder catheter. It is known that the ischiocavernosus muscle facilitates erection and that the bulbocavernosus muscle is involved in its maintenance. The reflux of blood from the corpora cavernosa is blocked by the contraction of the bulbocavernosus muscles that press on the deep dorsal vein of the penis. PFMT could increase ischiocavernosus and bulbocavernosus strength, endurance, and muscle coordination, but there is limited evidence that pelvic floor exercises (Fig. 8.2) relieve ED due to venous leakage and are a realistic alternative to surgery [20].

8.2 Biofeedback

Biofeedback is used in rehabilitation to facilitate normal movement patterns after injury. It is accounted as an important mind-body technique that involves controlling involuntary bodily functions. It emerged as a field of study in the 1960s, and since then, it has increasingly been used as a complementary or alternative way for treatments of symptoms in many clinical conditions and measurement of a target biomedical variable as heart rate function, respiration, blood pressure and flow, skin temperature, and disorders of muscle activity. To relay this target biomedical variable to the user, it includes two strategies: direct feedback as in the case of heart rate, where a numerical value is displayed on a wearable device such as a watch, or transformed feedback regarding the measured variable, where the measurements are used to control an adaptive auditory signal, visual display, or tactile feedback signals that can be perceived by the patient.

The biofeedback measurements which are frequently used in physical rehabilitation can be categorized as being either physiological or biomechanical [21]. The physiological systems of the body which can be measured to provide biofeedback are the neuromuscular system, the respiratory system, and the cardiovascular system, while biomechanical biofeedback involves measurements of movement, postural control, and force. Biofeedback may also be classified according to the type of signal used. EMG biofeedback is a method of retraining muscle by creating new feedback systems as a result of the conversion of myoelectrical signals in the muscle into visual and auditory signals. EMG biofeedback uses surface electrodes to detect a change in skeletal muscle activity, which is then feedback to the user usually by a visual or auditory signal. EMG biofeedback can be used to either increase activity in weak or paretic muscle or it can be used to facilitate a reduction in tone in a spastic one. Before or after radical prostatectomy, the use of this technique is indicated to treat alterations in muscle strength and muscle coordination, both during the acquisition phase of motor activity and during the improvement phase. This motor learning tool is also used when, upon request for contraction, agonist or antagonist muscles (adductors, gluteus) are activated, i.e., in the event of muscle incoordination, since it allows detection through surface electrodes. In this way, the subject learns to inhibit this activity. The technique includes the use of an anal electromyographic probe and it has no contraindications when used before or after radical prostatectomy.

8.2.1 Biofeedback for Urinary Dysfunction

There is strong evidence that, in addition to PFMT, biofeedback may provide intermediate and long-term benefits to men experiencing urinary incontinence after a prostatectomy, but the scientific evidence regarding the use of biofeedback in the treatment of post-prostatectomy urinary incontinence, in isolation or in addition to PFMT, are conflicting [22–24]. Certainly, biofeedback has significant advantages compared to other therapies used for the treatment of incontinence: It is a well-tolerated procedure, which can be carried out, after appropriate training, at home even without the support of the therapist and could be started within 1 year after the surgical procedures. It allows to perform special muscle movements to improve muscle strength, support the urinary tract, prevent urinary leakage, and improve urgency. However, EAU guidelines have pointed out that there is conflicting evidence as to whether adding biofeedback increases the efficacy of PFMT alone.

The use of BFB alone or associated with PFME/PFMT for post-prostatectomy urinary incontinence is considered in a systematic review by Hall et al. [8] which highlights discordant results with respect to the efficacy of PFME + BFB. The 3-month pooled analysis revealed significantly better results for PFMT than the control groups if PFMT included BFB but if no BFB was present, the effect became insignificant. The ICI states that the use of in-clinic BFB, in addition to home PFMT, should remain a therapist/individual decision based on economy and preference (grade of recommendation: B) [25]. In Kannan's review [26], the effect of PFMT + BFB on post-prostatectomy incontinence remains uncertain. The work of Sciarra et al. [22] suggests that a specific BFB program or the addition of ES to PFME significantly improves short-term outcomes (1- and 3-month intervals), both in terms of pad weight reduction and the recovery rate of the continence (without pads), when compared with the use of postoperatively assisted simple PFME or without a physiotherapist. Conversely, this advantage is not significant in long-term follow-up (6 and 12 months) although the results continue to be better by adding BF and/or ES to PFME.

These controversial results could be due to the fact that the effects of biofeedback are not immediate: The training results could be visible only after 6–8 weeks, and a high patient compliance is also required for them to become a real advantage in improving continence.

Furthermore, urinary incontinence often improves spontaneously within a few weeks after surgical procedures and, consequently, the possibility of finding significant results disappears and cannot be scientifically demonstrated.

However, what is important to underline is that biofeedback training does not only aim to strengthen the pelvic muscles but mainly influences functional disorders improving muscle coordination. For this reason, even if the short-term effects are not demonstrated, preoperative motor learning could improve the effects of postoperative rehabilitation; therefore, biofeedback could have a high clinical value and more attention should be paid to the use of the preoperative biofeedback courses in patients.

Actually, the use of the BF to assist PFMT is generally based on therapist or patient preference or on the availability of equipment in dedicated continence clinics.

8.2.2 Biofeedback for Bowel Dysfunction

Known experimental data allow us to state that biofeedback is effective in obtaining remission of fecal incontinence [27].

Fecal incontinence, the involuntary loss of solid or liquid stools, significantly worsens the quality of life of patients and places a significant burden on health-care providers and services. Pelvic radiotherapy is an important risk factor as it induces changes in the normal physiological functions of continence. Intestinal damage can be limited if radiation therapy for prostate cancer patients is given to a full urinary bladder. The full bladder has the potential to displace the small intestine out of radiation treatment regions and results in a reduction in small intestinal radiation dose and gastrointestinal toxicity. When present, intestinal damage can be treated with biofeedback, as usually happens in the management of fecal incontinence from other causes.

Biofeedback training is an established treatment modality for fecal incontinence; however, its role in post-radiotherapy patients for pelvic malignancies has yet to be established. The goal is to increase a patient's conscious control of the pathways that control defecation by reducing involuntary stool loss and defecation urgency.

It can be done in a variety of modalities, including balloon systems to facilitate patient awareness of rectal distension, ultrasound visualization of the anal sphincter and demonstration of the effects of a patient's exercises, and the use of anal manometric probes to teach the patient how to exercise the anal sphincter.

In general, patients are very interested in improving fecal continence, even more than urinary, and this significantly improves adherence to treatment.

8.2.3 Biofeedback for Erectile Dysfunction

The positive effects of biofeedback on erectile dysfunction are based on the theory that early penile circulation could speed up recovery by preventing corporal fibrosis and penile contracture.

Early rehabilitation care might accelerate local blood circulation to the penis in order to prevent corporal hypoxia and subsequent cavernosal fibrosis and to facilitate vascular and neural recovery.

Literature data are poor but allow us to state that patients undergoing biofeedback early experience more ease in solving ED later [28].

References

1. Hodges P, Stafford R, Coughlin GD, et al. Efficacy of a personalised pelvic floor muscle training programme on urinary incontinence after radical prostatectomy (MaTchUP): protocol for a randomised controlled trial. BMJ Open. 2019;9(5):e028288.
2. Strączyńska A, Weber-Rajek M, Strojek K, et al. The impact of pelvic floor muscle training on urinary incontinence in men after radical prostatectomy (RP)—a systematic review. Clin Interv Aging. 2019;14:1997–2005.
3. Stafford RE, Coughlin G, Lutton NJ, et al. Validity of estimation of pelvic floor muscle activity from transperineal ultrasound imaging in men. PLoS One. 2015;10:e0144342.
4. Kim YU, Lee DG, Ko YH. Pelvic floor muscle exercise with biofeedback helps regain urinary continence after robot-assisted radical prostatectomy. Yeungnam Univ J Med. 2021;38(1):39–46.
5. Filocamo MT, Li Marzi V, Del Popolo G, et al. Effectiveness of early pelvic floor rehabilitation treatment for post-prostatectomy incontinence. Eur Urol. 2005;48:734–8.
6. Wang W, Huang QM, Liu FP, et al. Effectiveness of preoperative pelvic floor muscle training for urinary incontinence after radical prostatectomy: a meta-analysis. BMC Urol. 2014;14:99–108.
7. Wu ML, Wang CS, Xiao Q, et al. The therapeutic effect of pelvic floor muscle exercise on urinary incontinence after radical prostatectomy: a meta-analysis. Asian J Androl. 2019;21:170–6.
8. Hall LM, Neumann P, Hodges PW. Do features of randomized controlled trials of pelvic floor muscle training for postprostatectomy urinary incontinence differentiate successful from unsuccessful patient outcomes? A systematic review with a series of meta-analyses. Neurourol Urodyn. 2020;39:533–46.
9. Mungovan SF, Carlsson SV, Gass GC, et al. Preoperative exercise interventions to optimize continence outcomes following radical prostatectomy. Nat Rev Urol. 2021;18:259–81.

10. Yokoyama T, Inoue M, Fujita O, et al. Preliminary results of the effect of extracorporeal magnetic stimulation on urinary incontinence after radical prostatectomy: a pilot study. Urol Int. 2005;74:224–8.
11. Goode PS, Burgio KL, Johnson TM 2nd, et al. Behavioral therapy with or without biofeedback and pelvic floor electrical stimulation for persistent postprostatectomy incontinence: a randomized controlled trial. JAMA. 2011;305:151–9.
12. Sandhu JS, Breyer B, Comiter C, et al. Incontinence after prostate treatment: AUA/SUFU guideline. J Urol. 2019;202:369–78.
13. Biroli A, Carone R. The prepubic stretching manoeuvre in post-prostatectomy incontinence rehabilitation. Urodinamica Neurourology Continence. 2002;12:267–8.
14. Bishoff JT, Motley G, Optenberg SA, et al. Incidence of fecal and urinary incontinence following radical perineal and retropubic prostatectomy in a national population. J Urol. 1998;160:454–8.
15. Nilssen SR, Mørkved S, Overgård M, et al. Does physiotherapist-guided pelvic floor muscle training increase the quality of life in patients after radical prostatectomy? A randomized clinical study. Scand J Urol Nephrol. 2012;46:397–404.
16. Milios JE, Ackland TR, Green DJ. Pelvic floor muscle training and erectile dysfunction in radical prostatectomy: a randomized controlled trial investigating a non-invasive addition to penile rehabilitation. Sex Med. 2020;8(3):414–21.
17. Schoentgen N, Califano G, Manfredi C, et al. Is it worth starting sexual rehabilitation before radical prostatectomy? Results from a systematic review of the literature. Front Surg. 2021;8:648345.
18. Nishikawa R, Honda M, Teraoka S, et al. Effects of nerve-sparing procedures on bowel function after robot-assisted radical prostatectomy: a longitudinal study. Int J Med Robot. 2020;16:1–10.
19. Saleh A, Abboudi H, Ghazal-Aswad M, et al. Management of erectile dysfunction post-radical prostatectomy. Res Rep Urol. 2015;7:19–33.
20. Overgard M, Angelsen A, Lydersen S, et al. Does physiotherapist-guided pelvic floor muscle training reduce urinary incontinence after radical prostatectomy? A randomised controlled trial. Eur Urol. 2008;54:438–48.
21. Floratos D, Sonke G, Rapidou C, et al. Biofeedback vs verbal feedback as learning tools for pelvic muscle exercises in the early management of urinary incontinence after radical prostatectomy. BJU Int. 2002;89:714–9.
22. Sciarra A, Viscuso P, Arditi A, et al. A biofeedback-guided programme or pelvic floor muscle electric stimulation can improve early recovery of urinary continence after radical prostatectomy: a meta-analysis and systematic review. Int J Clin Pract. 2021;75:e14208.
23. Ong TA, Khong SY, Ng KL, et al. Using the Vibrance Kegel device with pelvic floor muscle exercise for stress urinary incontinence: a randomized controlled pilot study. Urology. 2015;86:487–91.
24. Perez FSB, Rosa NC, da Rocha AF, et al. Effects of biofeedback in preventing urinary incontinence and erectile dysfunction after radical prostatectomy. Front Oncol. 2018;8:20–9.
25. Dumoulin C, Adewuyi T, Booth J, et al. Adult conservative management. In: Abrams P, Cardozo L, Wagg A, Wein A, editors. Incontinence: 6th international consultation on incontinence, Tokyo, September 2016, vol. 1. 6th ed. Bristol: International Continence Society (ICS) and International Consultation on Urological Diseases (ICUD).
26. Kannan P, Winser SJ, Fung B, et al. Effectiveness of pelvic floor muscle training alone and in combination with biofeedback, electrical stimulation, or both compared to control for urinary incontinence in men following prostatectomy: systematic review and meta-analysis. Phys Ther. 2018;98:932–45.
27. Raina R, Pahlajani G, Agarwal A, et al. Early penile rehabilitation following radical prostatectomy: Cleveland Clinic experience. Int J Impot Res. 2008;20:121–6.
28. Briganti A, Montorsi F. Penile rehabilitation after radical prostatectomy. Nat Clin Pract Urol. 2006;3:400–1.

External Devices for Urinary, Bowel, and Erectile Dysfunction

9

Giuseppina Gibertini, Roberta Robol, and Luisa De Palma

Incontinence aids should not be considered as an alternative to treatment, except in the most severe and unimprovable cases, but rather an additional and complementary support to treatment, aimed at facilitating the maintenance of a good quality of life until the problem has been solved.

Aids are not intended to "cure" incontinence but to help manage the problem to make it as tolerable and less disabling as possible.

In some cases, the use of aids, such as intermittent catheterization, is the optimal and permanent therapeutic solution.

The objectives of treatment with urinary incontinence aids are:

- To protect the skin of the genitals from the irritating action of urine and the aggression of moisture
- To protect clothing and bedding from sometimes irreversible damage
- To control the spread of bad odors and improve social life while preserving personal discretion and dignity

G. Gibertini (✉)
Neuro-Urology Unit, AOU Città della Salute e della Scienza, Torino, Italy
e-mail: ggibertini@cittadellasalute.to.it

R. Robol
Obstetric and Gynecology Unit, ASST Sette Laghi, Varese, Italy

L. De Palma
Physical, Rehabilitation Medicine and Spinal Cord Unit, Polyclinic of Bari, Bari, Italy

G. Lamberti, C. De Nunzio (eds.), *Bladder, Bowel and Sexual Dysfunctions Rehabilitation after Radical Prostatectomy*, Urodynamics, Neurourology and Pelvic Floor Dysfunctions, https://doi.org/10.1007/978-3-031-76341-0_9

Before recommending or procuring an aid, consideration must be given to its appropriateness for the individual case, taking into account various aspects such as:

- Gender
- Age
- The extent and frequency of leakages
- If the incontinence is only diurnal, only nocturnal, or persistent
- The condition of the skin
- The person's general condition (cognitive state, mobility, ability to self-manage, visual acuity, manual dexterity) in relation to the:
- Practical management of the aid
- The availability of the aid
- Treatment of waste

Incontinence aids are first divided into retention aids, that is, they supplement the inability to retain urine, and aids that remedy an inability to empty the bladder (catheters) that would result in the appearance of urine leakage as a result of urinary retention.

Retention aids include three groups:

- External urine collection systems
- Occlusive devices
- Absorbent products

Several urine collection systems are available:

The "urinary condom" (Fig. 9.1) is the most widely used in men for its convenience, cost-effectiveness, and easy disposal. It is a condom-shaped device connected to a urine collection bag. The condom must be hypoallergenic, transparent to better monitor the condition of the skin, liquid-proof, easy to put on and remove, nonirritating, and available in different sizes.

The condoms are commercially available in three materials:

1. Latex
2. Synthetic latex
3. Silicone

The fastening system can be internal, using an adhesive that makes the sheath adhere to the skin (double-sided adhesive strips, self-adhesive condoms, or condoms with glue applied separately), or external, using a tight-fitting band.

Its terminal end must be constructed so as not to fold over on itself. There are, however, complications associated with the use of these products, such as sudden loss of adherence resulting in urine leakage, especially during training, which may lead to abandonment of the aid, or dermatitis due to allergy or bacterial infection, ischemia and/or necrosis of the penile skin, urethral erosion, and increased incidence of urinary infections.

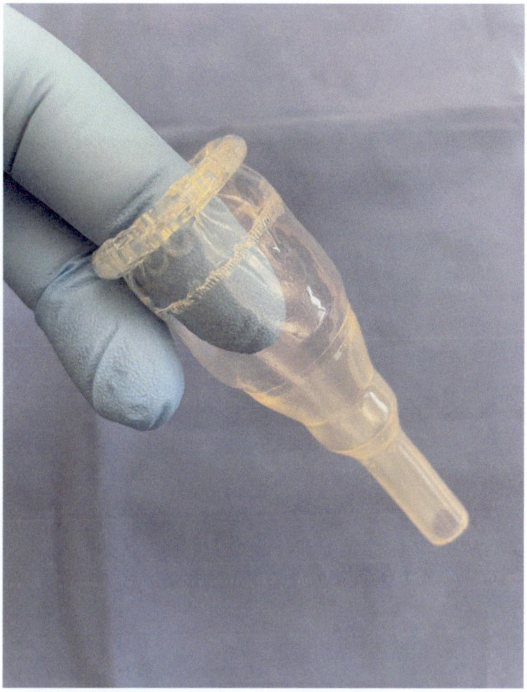

Fig. 9.1 Urinary condom

Care not to exert excessive pressure or traction on the penis is particularly important in patients with altered skin sensitivity.

A small or retractable penis or a redundant prepuce may limit its use. In some cases, prior circumcision is necessary.

The occlusive devices currently available are for male use only and prevent incontinence in some cases by allowing the bladder to fill. They are therefore recommended when it is necessary to prevent bladder deterioration due to insufficient filling.

The most commonly used are "penis clamps" (Fig. 9.2), which are applied to the penis to occlude the urethra. One type consists of an adjustable clamp with foam rubber-covered branches, which helps reduce trauma. It is washable, reusable, fairly effective, but nevertheless often not tolerated. It should be tightened as little as possible to achieve continence in order to avoid complications such as skin necrosis, urethral erosions, or especially abscesses, which are possible if it is worn for a long time. Another model is made of fabric and has a pad that presses on the urethra and is held in place by a Velcro strap (Fig. 9.3). It is smaller and lighter and therefore better tolerated but also less effective.

Absorbent products give a simple, fast, practical, and efficient response to the problems induced by incontinence and enable patients to regain the autonomy that is fundamental for the quality of life.

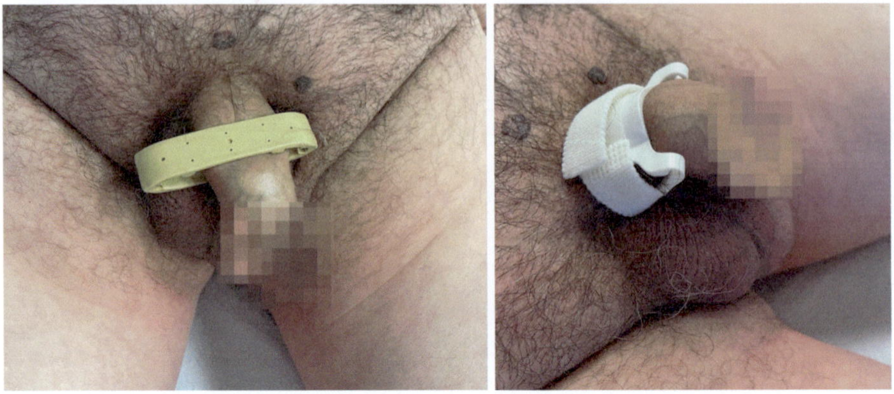

Fig. 9.2 Penis clamps

Fig. 9.3 Velcro strap

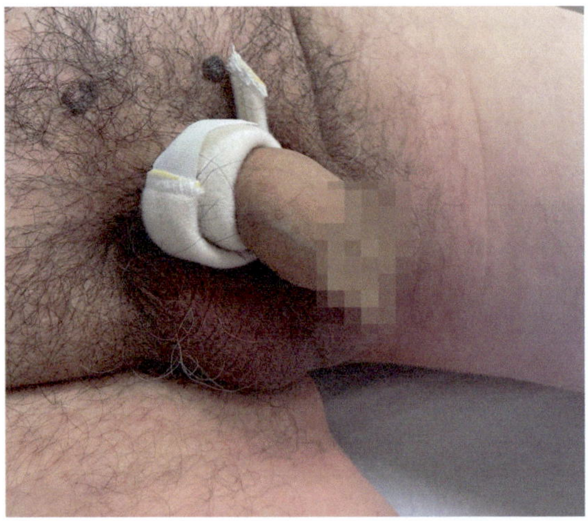

However, abuse, which can be induced by ease of use, should be avoided by avoiding their continued use on individuals for whom incontinence can be resolved with appropriate treatment and/or assistance.

They are the most commonly used and widespread aids, which have gradually become more comfortable and safe, thanks to the continuous innovations made by the industry.

They exist in many types and formats (Fig. 9.4), some more modern and innovative than others.

Having no particular contraindications per se, if used correctly, they are recommended whenever there is leakage that needs to be promptly absorbed to remove urine from the skin.

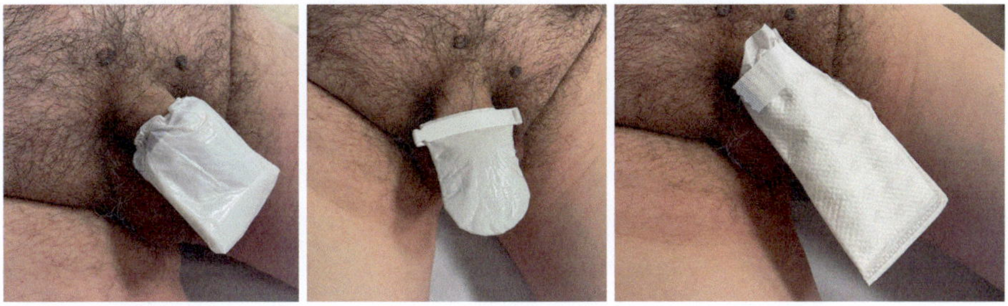

Fig. 9.4 Drip saver

In the case of severe incontinence that cannot be permanently resolved, choosing and using the "right" absorbent aid correctly is a decisive factor in promoting the recovery of continence (e.g., by facilitating "toilet training" in rehabilitation programs) or in delaying the loss of residual continence and autonomy as much as possible.

In addition to performing the primary functions of retention and dryness maintenance just described, which are clearly the most important, each absorbent pad should at the same time allow the achievement of other fundamental objectives such as:

- *Ease of use*: Positioning, removing, and disposing of the aid by the incontinent person or by those who assist them must be as easy and as fast as possible.
- *Comfort*: Understood as general comfort and absence of discomfort for those who wear the aid.
- *Discretion*: Especially for socially active people, the fact that the aid does not reveal its presence (reduced bulkiness, absence of rustling and smells) is of enormous importance in order not to affect the social sphere of the person and their self-esteem.
- *Respect for the environment*: Aids with a more modern and less bulky design, and with a longer service, generate less waste to be disposed of over time.

Overall, however, there is no such thing as the ideal or "the best" pad.

Depending on the situation and the specific needs of each incontinent person, it is possible and appropriate to identify the best solution for that case.

Since absorbent aids are devices for personal use, apart from some more general recommendations and selection criteria that we will set out below, the best criterion for assessment and choice is direct testing by the incontinent person, if necessary under the guidance and with the information support of those providing assistance.

The possibility and freedom to make an informed choice on a case-by-case basis is the best guarantee for an appropriate healthcare response.

10 Electrical Stimulation and Vacuum Device for Urinary, Bowel, and Erectile Dysfunction

Caterina Gruosso, Donatella Giraudo, Elena Bertolucci, and Luisa De Palma

10.1 Electrical Stimulation for Urinary, Bowel, and Erectile Dysfunction

The main trigger of incontinence after prostatectomy is probably secondary to sphincter damage caused by surgery to the prostate.

In the past years, it has been confirmed that the preservation of neuromuscular bundles may allow better recovery of urinary continence, and this finding confirmed that the damage may be secondary to a neurogenic dysfunction [1]. It has also been observed that detrusor overactivity may develop as an iatrogenic effect after surgery.

To date, the treatment of post-prostatectomy urinary incontinence is based on lifestyle modifications and therapeutic pelvic floor muscle training (PFMT), possibly in combination with biofeedback (BFB), electrostimulation (ES), extracorporeal magnetic stimulation, and the use of external devices in some cases [2].

Individual treatments or their combination have so far not demonstrated indisputable efficacy [3]. In general, ES is believed to inhibit detrusor contractions, thereby reducing the number of contractions and potentially increasing detrusor capacity, acting through two spinal reflexes that have the pudendal nerve endings as

C. Gruosso
Lecturer at Master's degree in pelvic floor rehabilitation, Tor Vergata University, Rome, Italy

D. Giraudo
Urology Department, San Raffaele Hosp. Ville Turro, Milan, Italy

E. Bertolucci (✉)
Physical, rehabilitation Medicine and Spinal Cord Unit, University Hospital Città della Salute e della Scienza, Torino, Italy

L. De Palma
Physical, Rehabilitation Medicine and Spinal Cord Unit, Polyclinic of Bari, Bari, Italy

G. Lamberti, C. De Nunzio (eds.), *Bladder, Bowel and Sexual Dysfunctions Rehabilitation after Radical Prostatectomy*, Urodynamics, Neurourology and Pelvic Floor Dysfunctions, https://doi.org/10.1007/978-3-031-76341-0_10

afferent pathways and the inhibitory neurons of the superior and inferior hypogastric plexuses as efferent pathways [4]. Similarly, ES can activate the skeletal muscles of the pelvic floor and it is therefore necessary, for it to be effective, to assume that at least partial pelvic floor innervation is present.

The mechanism of action is therefore twofold: an efferent stimulation, which determines a direct response of the different striated muscle components of the pelvic floor, and of the periurethral striated component [5], with a consequent reflex inhibition of the detrusor mediated by the sacral Onuf's nucleus (S2–S4 myelomeres), or a neuromodulating afferent stimulation on the detrusor-inhibiting reflexes [6].

Unlike therapeutic exercise, which can only evoke voluntary contraction, efferent stimulation is able to determine direct and reflexive responses and on the urethral and pelvic floor striated muscles [7, 8], thus increasing awareness of pelvic floor muscles, in a similar way to that obtained with BFB [3].

ES is believed to be most effective in patients who are initially unable to correctly identify and contract their pelvic floor muscles, with the assumption that its use may improve the outcome of exercise.

ES, along with exercise, has been shown to be effective in treating women with stress incontinence while the same combination in male urinary incontinence after radical prostatectomy needs further confirmation [9].

The literature describes two ways to administer ES after prostatectomy: the first via perineal surface electrodes for efferent and/or afferent stimulation and via penile surface electrodes (Fig. 10.1) for afferent stimulation, exploiting the unique sensory

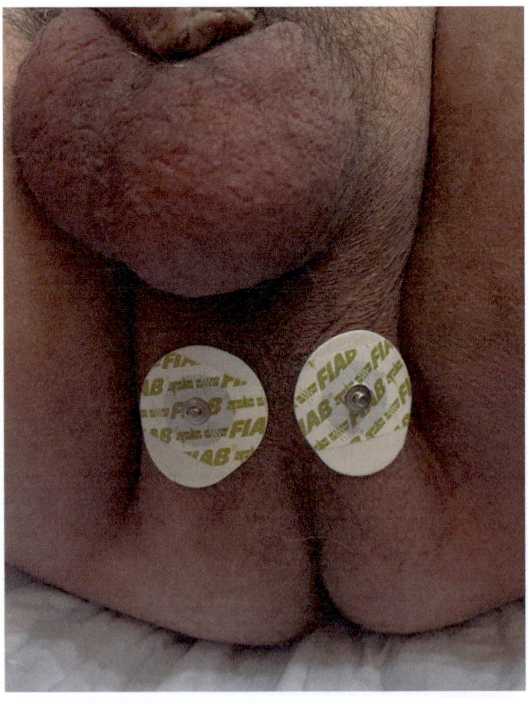

Fig. 10.1 Perineal surface electrodes for efferent and/or afferent stimulation

component of the dorsal nerve of the penis. The second method provides both efferent and afferent stimulation with the use of an anal probe, ideally shaped in such a way as to ensure stimulation above the pectinate line, so as to reduce the possible discomfort caused especially in the case of efferent stimulation.

Several randomized trials compared anal electrostimulation with sham stimulation [10–14] in incontinent patients after prostatectomy. ES was applied as the only treatment or, more frequently, as a treatment associated with therapeutic exercise, with a follow-up of 4–12 months after surgery, demonstrating greater benefits compared to controls. Two clinical trials, albeit with a limited number of study populations, have shown benefit with the use of ES combined with therapeutic exercise compared with sham treatment, but only in the first 6 months after surgery [9, 13]. The association with perineal ES with surface electrodes has also been shown to be more effective than therapeutic exercise alone [15, 16] or no treatment. Two studies [17, 18] have not confirmed these results. Studies are currently underway to demonstrate the similarity in effectiveness of ES with intracavitary electrodes and perineal ES with surface electrodes [19].

Other studies have, however, not confirmed that ES in combination with therapeutic exercise treatment [20, 21] or even alone can bring about further benefit [22].

To date, there is still a need for further studies on the efficacy of ES after radical prostatectomy in order to achieve a recovery of urinary continence.

10.1.1 Method of Administration

The efferent ES uses a sufficiently adequate electrical impulse to obtain the contraction of the muscles of the perineal plane: For the same duration of the stimulus, it is possible to obtain a greater recruitment by increasing the intensity (often, however, with the achievement of values that are poorly tolerated by the patient). With regard to the time factor, in males, it is confirmed that stimuli of greater duration (equal to or greater than 200 μs) preferentially stimulate the motor efferent nerve fibers, while stimuli of lesser duration excite the sensory afferent nerve fibers as a priority. The clinical assessment must guide the choice of the most appropriate frequencies according to the rehabilitation project. If the main objective is to improve the recruitment of the striated muscles of the pelvic floor in order to reduce iatrogenic surgical damage, suitable electrical impulse specifications should be chosen since different frequencies are able to selectively stimulate neurons innervating phasic muscle fibers (fast twitch) or tonic muscle fibers (slow twitch). The tonic fibers that must be stimulated in the case of reduced endurance are stimulated primarily by frequencies between 10 and 20 Hz, while when stimulating the phasic fibers for reduced proprioception, particularly in the early stages of rehabilitation treatment, frequencies between 30 and 50 Hz can be used, and only occasionally for more immediate awareness, frequencies of up to 80 Hz can be used. In summary, frequencies around 30 Hz with a duration of 250–300 μs seem able to activate the fibers of the pelvic floor with the main objective of increasing the recruitment of the same and electively the fast-twitch fibers. It is instead appropriate to use lower frequencies, around 5 Hz, in case the main objective is the stimulation of the smaller afferent fibers through the pudendal nerve, with duration of the stimulus around 150 μs. It is important when planning the session to identify the ratio between the duration of the stimulating current passage and the duration of the pause. A fundamental rule is a ratio of at least one to two between stimulation period and rest period in order not to fatigue the affected muscle. The currents used in the treatment are symmetrical bipolar zero resultant waves: This is the only type that avoids the annoying polarizing effects of monopolar current. Since it is not possible to determine the crown of both the perineal musculature, the optimal stimulation intensity values can only be determined on the basis of the subjective perception of the stimulus passage or, rather, on the basis of the visual detection of the perineal contraction. The rise of the pelvic floor and the central fibrous nucleus of the perineum must be verified in order to be certain that an effective current is being used.

10.1.2 ES in Post-prostatectomy Erectile Dysfunction

To date, there is insufficient data in the literature to support the use of electrical stimulation to treat post-radical prostatectomy erectile dysfunction (ED) [23]. Two studies have highlighted the efficacy of surface ES as the only treatment with a cure rate between 10% and 23% [24, 25]. The association of anal ES with PFMT was studied using pulses of 35 Hz with a duration of 1 ms, twice weekly for 7 weeks; however, no significant results on ED were observed, although the authors assume that the persistence of urinary incontinence was the cause of limitation in sexual activity [22]. On the other hand, another study showed a benefit in combined treatment with ES (50 Hz frequency and 600 μs pulse duration) and PFMT [26]. In treatment with surface ES, a St. Mark's electrode can be used (Fig. 10.2), employing a bipolar technique, to bilaterally obtain the selective contraction of the ischiocavernosus muscle and the bulbospongiosus muscle.

10.2 Vacuum Device for Erectile Dysfunction

Physiological erectile function requires the coexistence and organization of several regulatory systems that are under hormonal, psychological, cavernous, neurological, and vascular influence. An impairment of even just one of these factors is sufficient to cause erectile dysfunction (ED). Often, the dysfunction sets in with a combination of these factors [27].

Several options are available for managing ED, including different types of treatment: oral phosphodiesterase type 5 inhibitors (PDE5i), intracavernous injections (ICI), intraurethral alprostadil (MUSE), and vacuum devices (VED) or combination therapies [28]. The proposed rationale for rehabilitation essentially consists of two strategies: preventing hypoxia to the corpora cavernosa and thereby reducing cavernous fibrosis, in the absence of spontaneous erections throughout the period of neurapraxia, and attempting to maintain smooth muscle integrity, potentially

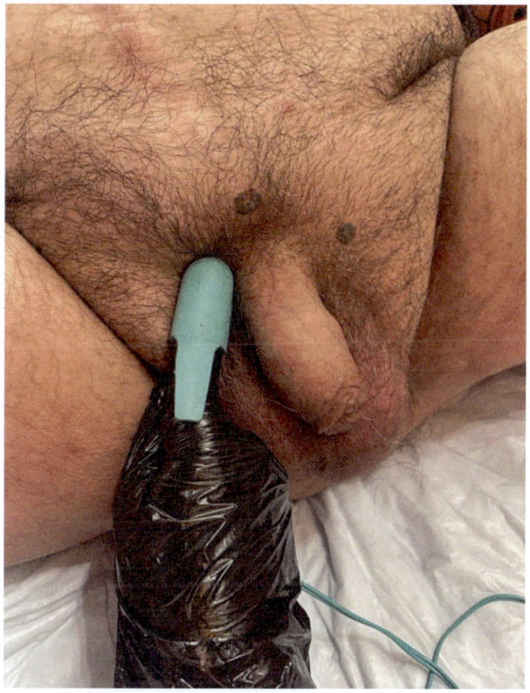

Fig. 10.2 Selective electrostimulation of ischiocavernosus muscle for erectile dysfunction

increasing the likelihood of preserving erectile function. In fact, the fibrotic changes that occur throughout the period of hypoxia due to the lack of spontaneous erections can be irreversible and lead to long-term ED [29]. The first clinical use of a prototype, with the application of vacuum technology, for the treatment of erectile dysfunction was used in 1874 by Dr. John King, but it was only after 1917 that Dr. Otto Lederer combined vacuum and compression to produce a device suitable for maintaining an erection achieved with vacuum. The first medically relevant device was taken from Dr. Lederer's model, developed and attributed to the Georgian entrepreneur Geddings D. Osbon in 1960. He is said to have used, studied, and disseminated it for over 20 years and finally obtained permission to market it by the US Food and Drug Administration in 1982 as a prescription device for the treatment of erectile dysfunction. Many models of the VED are currently on the market but all share the same basic mechanics since its inception. The VED consists of a transparent plastic cylinder with the end closed by a vacuum pump that can be operated by hand or can be powered by a battery-powered electric motor. The patient is generally advised to lubricate the entire penile shaft with a water-soluble lubricant and then insert the penis into the cylinder, placing the base of the same very tightly at the base of the penis to create an airtight seal. With one hand, hold the cylinder at the base of the penis while using the other hand to operate the manual pump or activate the switch of the electric pump. The VED uses negative pressure (100–225 mmHg) to dilate the sinusoids and increase blood flow to the corpora cavernosa, causing an erection.

This induced erection may initially involve only the most proximal tissues, so it is recommended to release the internal cylinder pressure and then start pumping again until the entire penile shaft is erect. The repeated action of blood engorgement and detumescence using the VED mimics normal physiological vascular function, creating a sort of tissue engorgement training. Once the necessary turgor has been achieved, the VED can also be used with an external constriction ring that is passed from the base of the device to the base of the penis to prevent the outflow of blood. With the mechanical maintenance of this erection, achieved by air vacuum and engorgement of all the tissues of the penis, the patient can attempt intercourse with penetration. In this case, we refer to a vacuum constriction device (VCD) [30]. The time required for an adequate erection can range from 30 s to 7 min, and this is related to the manual ability of the patient or his partner. However, as the blood that flows to the penis is non-arterious blood, as in a physiological erection, although some authors [31] argue that there is a percentage share of arterial blood, the use of the constriction ring prevents venous return, creating hypoxia in the tissues. In fact, manufacturers generally recommend that the ring should not remain in place for more than 30 min to avoid ischemic injury to the penis [32]. The benefits of using the VCD with the constriction ring are many, as we have seen, especially in terms of the possible resumption of sexual intercourse and the impact on the quality of life: It is quick to use. It can be incorporated in the foreplay to sexual intercourse with more spontaneous gestures than other techniques. It is less invasive than other techniques. It is cheap, i.e., affordable given the one-off purchase with a good duration of more than 5 years. It has few contraindications. Complications, in fact, are considered minor: pain related to the ring or vacuum, which is however usually self-limiting. The ring may cause ejaculatory discomfort or secondary ejaculatory inability due to urethral constriction. The penis may appear cold and cyanotic gray/bluish which could create discomfort for both partners. Since it is not a true erection, the penis points downward and its base presents a certain flaccidity near the ring, the root of the penis cannot be congested from within the perineum, and this makes the retention of the penis in the vagina unstable, forcing partners to continuous manipulation during intercourse. The penis may present some numbness or bruising and petechiae, hemorrhagic events, and priapism [33]. The use of VED without a constriction ring (Fig. 10.3) is a primary application in penile rehabilitation as it is able to supply blood flow to the tissues even in the presence of nerve injury. This increased blood flow or tumescence in the penis shaft can reduce the risk or even intervene in the fibrotic changes that occur after radical prostatectomy surgery. Given its low complication rate [34], high satisfaction and efficacy rate [35], and high tolerability and safety [36], the use of VED, without the constriction ring, is an ideal and primary method to adopt in rehabilitation protocols after radical prostatectomy, resulting in a 60% improvement in spontaneous erections, as well as a significant improvement in International Index of Erectile Function (IIEF) scores, especially when used early after surgery [37]. Furthermore, the use of VED can help prevent penile shrinkage in both length and girth in patients undergoing permanent treatment for prostate cancer [38]. Penile rehabilitation, therefore, is defined as a treatment to improve the restoration of the natural mechanics of the penis, i.e., in a

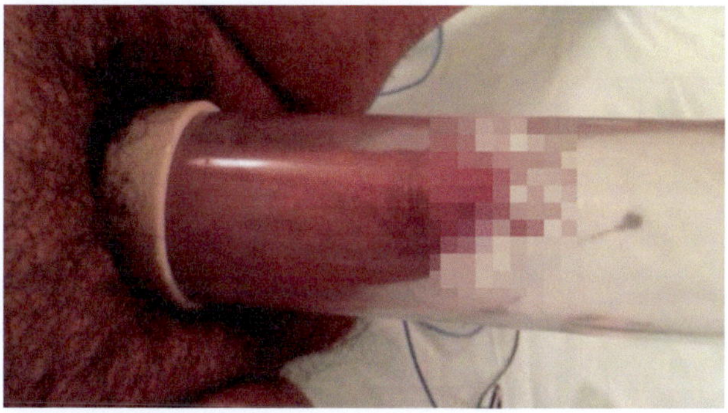

Fig. 10.3 Vacuum device without a constriction ring for penile rehabilitation

recovery of spontaneous erectile function. A survey, conducted during the American Urological Association (AUA) annual meeting involving 618 urologists, showed that rehabilitation is a common practice and that the most commonly used strategy is the regular use of phosphodiesterase type 5 inhibitors (PDE5I), as the primary strategy, followed by the vacuum erection device (VED). Although there is currently no consensus on a single optimal protocol, vacuum device rehabilitation is widely applied in clinical practice. The daily use of the VED with progressive erection and detumescence action is generally recommended continuously for at least 15–20 min [39].

References

1. Kaiho Y, Nakagawa H, Ikeda Y, et al. Intraoperative electrophysiological confirmation of urinary continence after radical prostatectomy. J Urol. 2005;173:1139–42.
2. Mottet N, Cornford P, van den Bergh R, et al. EAU-EANM-ESTRO-ESUR-ISUP-SIOG guidelines on prostate cancer. Arnhem: EAU Guidelines Office; 2022.
3. Anderson CA, Omar MI, Campbell SE, et al. Conservative management for postprostatectomy urinary incontinence. Cochrane Database Syst Rev. 2015;1(1):CD001843.
4. Fall M. Does electrostimulation cure urinary incontinence? J Urol. 1984;131:664–7.
5. Berghmans B, Hendriks E, Bernards A, et al. Electrical stimulation with non-implanted electrodes for urinary incontinence in men. Cochrane Database Syst Rev. 2013;(6):CD001202.
6. Vodusek DB, Janko M, Lokar J. Direct and reflex responses in perineal muscles on electrical stimulation. J Neurol Neurosurg Psychiatry. 1983;46:67–71.
7. Yamanishi T, Kamai T, Yoshida K. Neuromodulation for the treatment of urinary incontinence. Int J Urol. 2008;15:665–72.
8. Walsh IK, Johnston RS, Keane PF. Transcutaneous sacral neurostimulation for irritative voiding dysfunction. Eur Urol. 1999;35:192–9.
9. Yamanishi T, Mizuno T, Watanabe M, et al. Randomized, placebo controlled study of electrical stimulation with pelvic floor muscle training for severe urinary incontinence after radical prostatectomy. J Urol. 2010;184:2007–12.
10. Van Kampen M, De Weerdt W, Van Poppel H, et al. Effect of pelvic-floor re-education on duration and degree of incontinence after radical prostatectomy: a randomised controlled trial. Lancet. 2000;355:98–102.
11. Gomes CS, Pedriali FR, Urbano MR, et al. The effects of Pilates method on pelvic floor muscle strength in patients with postprostatectomy urinary incontinence: a randomized clinical trial. Neurourol Urodyn. 2018;37:346–53.

12. Pedriali FR, Gomes CS, Soares L, et al. Is Pilates as effective as conventional pelvic floor muscle exercises in the conservative treatment of post-prostatectomy urinary incontinence? A randomised controlled trial: is Pilates as effective as conventional pelvic. Neurourol Urodyn. 2016;35:615–21.
13. Mariotti G, Sciarra A, Gentilucci A, et al. Early recovery of urinary continence after radical prostatectomy using early pelvic floor electrical stimulation and biofeedback associated treatment. J Urol. 2009;181:1788–93.
14. Kannan P, Winser SJ, Fung B, et al. Effectiveness of pelvic floor muscle training alone and in combination with biofeedback, electrical stimulation, or both compared to control for urinary incontinence in men following prostatectomy: systematic review and meta-analysis. Phys Ther. 2018;98:932–45.
15. Hoffmann W, Liedke S, Dombo O, et al. Electrostimulation in therapy of postoperative urinary incontinence. Therapeutic value for quality of life. Urol A. 2005;44:33–40.
16. Yıldız N, Çelen S, Özlülerden Y, et al. Efficacy of perineal electrical stimulation in men with urinary incontinence after radical prostatectomy. A prospective randomized controlled trial. Neurourol Urodyn. 2023;42:340–8.
17. Moore KN, Griffiths D, Hughton A. Urinary incontinence after radical prostatectomy: a randomized controlled trial comparing pelvic muscle exercises with or without electrical stimulation. BJU Int. 1999;83:57–65.
18. Wille S, Sobottka A, Heidenreich A, et al. Pelvic floor exercises, electrical stimulation and biofeedback after radical prostatectomy: results of a prospective randomized trial. J Urol. 2003;170:490–3.
19. Pané-Alemany R, Ramírez-García I, Kauffmann S, et al. Efficacy of transcutaneous perineal electrostimulation versus intracavitary anal electrostimulation in the treatment of urinary incontinence after a radical prostatectomy: randomized controlled trial. Neurourol Urodyn. 2021;40:1761–9.
20. Goode PS, Burgio KL, Johnson TM, et al. Behavioral therapy with or without biofeedback and pelvic floor electrical stimulation for persistent postprostatectomy incontinence: a randomized controlled trial. JAMA. 2011;305:151–9.
21. Zhu YP, Yao XD, Zhang SL, et al. Pelvic floor electrical stimulation for postprostatectomy urinary incontinence: a meta-analysis. Urology. 2012;79:552–5.
22. Laurienzo CE, Magnabosco WJ, Jabur F, et al. Pelvic floor muscle training and electrical stimulation as rehabilitation after radical prostatectomy: a randomized controlled trial. J Phys Ther Sci. 2018;30:825–31.
23. Feng D, Tang C, Liu S, et al. Current management strategy of treating patients with erectile dysfunction after radical prostatectomy: a systematic review and meta-analysis. Int J Impot Res. 2022;34:18–36.
24. Stief CG, Weller E, Noack T, et al. Functional electromyostimulation of the corpus cavernosum penis--preliminary results of a novel therapeutic option for erectile dysfunction. World J Urol. 1995;13:243–7.
25. Derouet H, Nolden W, Jost WH, et al. Treatment of erectile dysfunction by an external ischiocavernous muscle stimulator. Eur Urol. 1998;34:355–9.
26. Geraerts I, Van Poppel H, Devoogdt N, et al. Pelvic floor muscle training for erectile dysfunction and climacturia 1 year after nerve sparing radical prostatectomy: a randomized controlled trial. Int J Impot Res. 2016;28:9–13.
27. Sáenz de Tejada I, Angulo J, Cellek S, González-Cadavid N, et al. Physiology of erectile function. J Sex Med. 2004;1:254–65.
28. Raina R, Pahlajani G, Agarwal A, et al. Long-term potency after early use of a vacuum erection device following radical prostatectomy. BJU Int. 2010;106:1719–22.
29. Raina R, Agarwal A, Zippe CD. Management of erectile dysfunction after radical prostatectomy. Urology. 2005;66:923–9.
30. Oakley N, Moore KT. Vacuum devices in erectile dysfunction: indications and efficacy. Br J Urol. 1998;82:673–81.

31. Broderick G, McGahan J, Stone A, et al. The hemodynamics of vacuum constriction erections: assessment by color Doppler ultrasound. J Urol. 1992;147:57–61.
32. Yuan J, Hoang AN, Romero CA, et al. Vacuum therapy in erectile dysfunction—science and clinical evidence. Int J Impot Res. 2010;22:211–9.
33. Lehrfeld T, Lee DI. The role of vacuum erection devices in penile rehabilitation after radical prostatectomy. Int J Impot Res. 2009;21:158–64.
34. Ganem JP, Lucey DT, Janosko EO, et al. Unusual complications of the vacuum erection device. Urology. 1998;51:627–31.
35. Albaugh JA. Addressing and managing erectile dysfunction after prostatectomy for prostate cancer. Urol Nurs. 2010;30:167–77.
36. Lin H, Wang R. The science of vacuum erectile device in penile rehabilitation after radical prostatectomy. Transl Androl Urol. 2013;2:61–6.
37. Köhler TS, Pedro R, Hendlin K, et al. A pilot study on the early use of the vacuum erection device after radical retropubic prostatectomy. BJU Int. 2007;100:858–62.
38. Dalkin BL, Christopher BA. Preservation of penile length after radical prostatectomy: early intervention with a vacuum erection device. Int J Impot Res. 2007;19:501–4.
39. Tal R, Teloken P, Mulhall JP. Erectile function rehabilitation after radical prostatectomy: practice patterns among AUA members. J Sex Med. 2011;8:2370–6.

Questionnaires and PROs for Urinary, Bowel, and Erectile Dysfunction After a Radical Prostatectomy

11

Cosimo De Nunzio, Giorgia Tema, Nicola Ghezzo, Antonio Testa, Noemi Deanesi, Gianluigi Raso, and Francesco Esperto

11.1 Introduction

Patients treated with radical prostatectomy (RP) face many postoperative challenges, from initial concerns such as wound healing to longer-term concerns, such as regaining sexual and bowel function and urinary control [1, 2]. Knowledge of the adverse events of different management options is fundamental to take informed treatment decisions, considering that the survival benefit is uncertain, especially in men with favorable-risk prostate cancer (PCa) [3]. Without efficient and structured tool to collect such parameter, physicians would be unable to collect the practices-specific outcomes information needed to offer adequate counseling. Reliable and efficient measures of function, bother, and mediating variables are necessary to identify the processes that foster successful adaptation to treatment complications. Ideally, such measures should be quickly and easily administered and suitable for use in multiple settings [4].

The adverse effects of treatments for localized disease can negatively impact quality of life (QoL) [5]. The physician attempting to discuss quality of life issues with prostate cancer patients in a realistic yet reassuring way is faced with a daunting task.

C. De Nunzio (✉)
Faculty of Psychology and Medicine, Urology Unit, Sapienza University of Rome, Sant'Andrea Hospital, Rome, Italy
e-mail: cosimo.denunzio@uniroma1.it

G. Tema · N. Ghezzo
Azienda Ospedaliera Universitaria Sant'Andrea, Rome, Italy
e-mail: gtema@osepdalesantandrea.it; nicola.ghezzo@uniroma1.it

A. Testa · N. Deanesi · G. Raso · F. Esperto
Fondazione Policlinico Universitario Campus Bio-Medico, Università Campus Bio-Medico di Roma, Rome, Italy

G. Lamberti, C. De Nunzio (eds.), *Bladder, Bowel and Sexual Dysfunctions Rehabilitation after Radical Prostatectomy*, Urodynamics, Neurourology and Pelvic Floor Dysfunctions, https://doi.org/10.1007/978-3-031-76341-0_11

Clinicians/investigators must be able to rigorously assess quality of life-related outcomes experienced by patients, allowing to effectively incorporate quality of life considerations into treatment decisions. Accurate evaluation of such outcomes allows to supply a more appropriate risk estimates for complications and facilitates clinicians to better inform their patients of how and to what extent treatment complications are likely to affect their lives [4, 6].

Several questionnaires are commonly used in post-RP management for the purpose of providing patient-directed assessments of symptoms. The benefits of patient-reported symptoms and outcomes include improved physician-patient communication and increased sensitivity in identifying dysfunction and provide a standardized method for assessing interventions and characterizing health at the population level [7, 8]. Moreover, many of these tools can also be adopted in the preoperative setting to determine baseline symptoms and functioning, making post-RP results more informative [1].

Patient-reported outcomes (PROs) are being used more and more over the time. As the 2023 EAU guidelines states, for quality control, and in order to help the patient in choosing the optimal treatment for him, it is essential that the functional outcomes of any treatment given are measured and registered by validated and reproducible methods. In order to address side effects and their impact of QoL, specific tools or "patient-reported outcome measures" (PROMs) have been developed and validated for men with PCa. These questionnaires assess common issues after PCa diagnosis and treatment and generate scores which reflect the impact on perceptions of HRQoL [9].

A patient-reported outcome (PRO) is a report that comes directly from the patient about the status of a health condition without amendment or interpretation of the response by a clinician or anyone else. PROs are self-reported through a wide variety of instruments known as patient-reported outcome measures (PROMs). Capturing a wide range of experiences longitudinally, PROMs are increasingly utilized tools [10].

Patients' reports of symptoms, function, and health-related quality of life (HRQL) or overall quality of life (QoL) provide significant data on the impact that health problems and related treatments have on patients' lives [11, 12].

The concept of QoL is subjective; however, in cancer cohorts, specific tools or patient-reported outcome measures (PROMs) have been developed and validated. These questionnaires assess common issues that affect men after PCa diagnosis and treatment and generate scores which reflect the impact on perceptions of health-related quality of life (HRQL) [3, 5].

HRQL focuses on the perceived impact (from the patient's perspective) of physical, mental, and social domains of health. HRQL is focused not exclusively on "how much symptom" the patient has but also on the level of bothering and concerning this symptom produces on the patient [13]. The performance of these instruments is often expressed in terms of reliability (the extent to which an instrument is free from error), validity (the extent to which it measures what it aims to measure), and responsiveness (the ability to detect clinically important changes over time) [12].

Over time, the number of different general HRQoL and disease-specific HRQoL questionnaires has increased tremendously, with a recent systematic review revealing 298 different questionnaires for prostate cancer. For this reason, it is important for clinicians who participate in PCa patients' management to grasp the characteristics and differences of the most widely used and validated general, cancer-specific, and prostate cancer-specific HRQoL questionnaires [1, 14].

A criticism of questionnaires may be related to cultural and language adaptations, such as the use of clinical terminology that patients may not comprehend, the real ability to detect a change in a patient's condition, and whether the change is meaningful to the patient (e.g., the severity of incontinence may vary according to lifestyle, age, job, and social conditions). Questionnaires are perceived by many to be too complicated for clinical practice.

However, it is important to promote the wider use of questionnaires to standardize the assessment of postoperative functional outcomes and its impact on patients' lives to facilitate communication in clinical practice and clinical research [15–17].

11.2 Urinary Dysfunction

Over the past decades, important improvements in surgical techniques have been made, but urinary incontinence (UI) is still not uncommon after radical prostatectomy (RP) and may dramatically worsen the quality of life of a patient who has been successfully cured of prostate cancer [16]. It usually appears immediately after the operation, but continence recovers partially or fully during the first months. Unfortunately, UI will be a lifetime problem for some patients.

The occurrence of UI after radical prostatectomy may depend on several factors including the definition of UI, the methodology used to assess continence, the time of follow-up, and, most importantly, the subjective evaluation of continence status by the patient. The last one can result being largely different between patients. For instance, while one is satisfied with his continence status even if required two pads per day, the other one is severely bothered by losing a drop during a physical effort. For this reason an objective evaluation of post-RP UI is fundamental not only to properly evaluate incontinence itself but also to evaluate the outcomes of new surgical techniques or postoperative treatments to improve continence recovery [16, 18].

Systematic reviews have documented complication rates after RALP and can be compared with contemporaneous reports after RRP. From these reports, the mean continence rates at 12 months were 89–100% for patients treated with RALP and 80–97% for patients treated with RRP. A prospective controlled non-randomized trial of patients undergoing RP in 14 centers using RALP or RRP demonstrated that at 12 months after RALP, 21.3% were incontinent, as were 20.2% after RRP. The unadjusted OR was 1.08 (95% CI: 0.87–1.34). Further follow-up demonstrates similar functional outcomes with both techniques at 24 months [9].

Stress UI (SUI) is the most common type of incontinence reported after RP, while urge incontinence (UUI) has only a minor impact, but daily pad use and 24-h pad weight test cannot distinguish between the two types. Urodynamic studies are useful for evaluating the pattern of UI; however, it is invasive and complicated [19]. The 2022 AUA guidelines on incontinence after prostate treatment state that "clinicians should evaluate patients with incontinence after prostate treatment with history, physical exam, and appropriate diagnostic modalities to categorize type and severity of incontinence and degree of bother" [20].

The first widely recognized urinary function questionnaire is the International Prostate Symptom Score (IPSS) [21]. Published in 1992, the IPSS was originally developed and validated to assess treatment in men with benign prostatic hyperplasia (BPH). Given the formal recommendation for its clinical utilization in the international guidelines, IPSS is nowadays one of the most commonly used questionnaires in this setting, explaining its familiarity among urologists [22].

It is favored for its simple scoring, minimal time commitment, and established cutoffs for symptom severity [23]. It is an 8-question Likert scale device: 4 questions about voiding symptoms, 3 questions about storage symptoms, and 1 QoL item.

Even if it represents a valid tool for the post-RP population, the IPSS does not provide any urinary incontinence information. At the moment, it has not been independently validated in post-RP patients; it is still commonly used to evaluate urinary function recovery after the intervention [24–26].

The International Consultation on Incontinence Questionnaire (ICIQ) has been developed to provide a simple, brief, and robust questionnaire to assess the symptoms and impact of incontinence that could be used universally in clinical practice and research. This is particularly important if it is to be used to monitor the status of patients' symptoms over time and to detect changes in the level and impact of patients' symptoms following various treatments [27]. Finally, a simple scoring system has been developed that is suitable, is scientifically justified, and demonstrates adequate psychometric properties [28].

The International Consultation on Incontinence Questionnaire-Short Form (ICIQ-SF) is a simple questionnaire for evaluating UI after RP, including a subjective UI evaluation and the pattern of UI [29]. Sponsored by the World Health Organization, the International Consultation on Incontinence aimed to develop a modular, universally accepted incontinence questionnaire for use across international populations, both for clinical practice and research. The initial product of this work was the development of the ICIQ Short Form Questionnaire for urinary incontinence (the ICIQ-UI Short Form). Developed in 2004, it is a brief 4-question Likert scale device validated in patients with incontinence and is currently available in over 60 languages [30]. To explore further urinary symptoms, including nocturia, overactive bladder, and sexual matters related to urinary symptoms, an additional module questionnaire, composed by 22 different ICIQ items, was produced.

As such, the ICIQ may be useful for clinicians and researchers aiming to subcategorize post-RP patients' symptoms [1].

In recent years, other questionnaires were developed to better define and evaluate UI, like the M-ISI questionnaire. This is a new 10-item questionnaire that was created to be able to discern type (SUI, UUI, or both), severity, and bother attributable to UI. It is psychometrically robust and has proven validity and reliability, and it can be easily administrated and possesses the robust psychometric criteria necessary for a research tool. Unlike other UI questionnaires, the M-ISI covers different aspects of UI that are essential for patient care and for research. For example, there are many questionnaires for UI that focus on quality of life issues (including severity and impact) but that neglect type of urinary incontinence. On the other hand, even if it represent a valid tool to evaluate UI after RP, it has been developed studying a general population, composed of men and women, and it's not validated after RP [31] (Table 11.1).

Table 11.1 Questionnaires and PROs for urinary function

Questionnaire	Authors	Domains	Response options	Scoring	Target population	Administration
IPSS	Barry et al. [21]	Four questions about voiding symptoms, three questions about storage symptoms, and one QoL item	0–5 Likert scale and one 0–10 Likert scale	Scoring system based on summary of items	Assessment of therapy in patients with prostatic symptoms (validated for BPH)	Self-administrated
International Consultation on Incontinence Questionnaire (ICIQ)	Abrams et al. [30]	Frequency and amount of leakages, bother, protections used, and interference with everyday/social/sex life	Multiple options with scores and one 0–10 points Likert scale	Scoring system based on summary of items	Patients with urinary leak	Self-administrated
International Consultation on Incontinence Questionnaire-Short Form (ICIQ-SF)	Kazuaki M. et al. [29]	Frequency and amount of leakages and everyday life impact	Multiple options with score and one 0–10 points Likert scale	Items 3–5 summed	Patients with urinary leak	Self-administrated
Michigan Incontinence Symptom Index (M-ISI)	A. M Suskind et al. [31]	Frequency of leakages (1–6), use of protection (7–8), and limitations and bother (9–10)	0–4 points Likert scale	Items 1–8 scores summed = total severity score; items 9–10 scores summed = total bother score	Patients with urinary leak	Self-administrated

11.3 Sexual Dysfunction

Sexual function is determined by different aspects: sexual desire, penile ability for erection, achievement of orgasm, frequency of intercourse, and other aspects. At the age of 50–80 years, sexual desire, erection capacity, and orgasm pleasure decreases naturally in 50–70% of men, causing enormous distress for them and their sexual partners [32]. Reports on sexual function in men after RP show large variability with regard to ability to gain erection. Until the introduction of nerve-sparing concepts, almost all men showed no regain of sexual function after surgery. But even when the anatomical integrity of the nerves seems to have been preserved, various categories of factors have been demonstrated to affect the recovery of potency, like comorbidities (diabetes, hypertension, arterial insufficiency, or even the patient's age itself) and surgeon's ability [33].

Although new surgical strategies as nerve-sparing surgery (NSS) and preservation of accessory pudendal artery were introduced to preserve erectile function, a rate of postoperative erectile dysfunction (ED) ranging between 25% and 75% has been reported in the literature.

A 2016 systematic review and meta-analysis included two small RCTs comparing RARP versus laparoscopic RP (LRP). The results suggested higher rates of return of erectile function (RR: 1.51, 95% CI: 1.19–1.92) in the RARP group. However, a Cochrane review comparing either RARP or LRP versus open RP included two RCTs and found no significant differences between the comparisons for oncological, urinary, and sexual function outcomes.

Erectile dysfunction at 12 months was observed in 70.4% after RALP and 74.7% after RRP. The unadjusted OR was 0.81 (95% CI: 0.66–0.98).

Although the most common postoperative complication after RP is ED, other sexual dysfunction as dry ejaculation, which always occurs with removal of the prostate, changes in the quality of orgasm and occasional pain on orgasm have been reported. Men also complain of loss of penile length (3.73%, 19/510 men) [9].

Due to the absence of a standardized methodology, the evaluation of erectile function has always been difficult, if not impossible. Because of the lack of a validated questionnaire, authors have used different instruments in order to estimate sexual function [33].

The first questionnaire developed for the evaluation of erectile function (EF) was the International Index of Erectile Function (IIEF-15). Developed in 1997, it is a 15-question device that established a framework for questionnaires in this space [34]. However, the IIEF-15 lacks distinct cutoffs for moderate and severe ED and imparts little information on sexual domains outside of erection.

The next evolution of the IIEF-15, published in 1999, was the International Index of Erectile Function 5 (IIEF-5), an abridged version of the IIEF-15 commonly referred to as the Sexual Health Inventory for MEN (SHIM). Advantages of the IIEF-5/SHIM questionnaire compared to the IIEF-15 include its abbreviated structure (5 vs. 15 items) and distinct cutoffs for severe ED and normal (<8 and >21, respectively). However, similar to the IIEF-15, the IIEF-5/SHIM is validated in heterosexual men and has a 6-month recall period, limiting its utility for prospective, long-term follow-up of erectile function [1, 35].

Departing from the IIEF framework, the Male Sex Health Questionnaire (MSHQ) is a 25-item questionnaire that was developed to globally assess male sexual function [36]. The MSHQ expands beyond the IIEF's focus on erectile function and includes questions about erection quality, ejaculatory function, orgasmic dysfunction, and overall sexual satisfaction [1, 37].

In contrast to multi-question devices, the Erection Hardness Score and Percent Full Erection questionnaires are validated, single-item devices relating to a patient's perceived degree of erectile rigidity. The Erection Hardness Score (EHS) was developed in 2007 and asks patients "How would you rate the hardness of your erection?" with a corresponding 5-item response scale ranging from "0: penis does not enlarge" to "4: penis is completely hard and fully rigid" [38]. The most obvious criticism of the EHS is its narrow, simplistic view of erectile function, based exclusively on perceived erectile rigidity, which may overlook other domains of normal erectile function, such as maintenance of erection and satisfaction [37].

An analogue tool, but different in execution, is represented by the Percent Full Erection (PFE): This scale asks the patient to report patient-reported fullness he is able to "achieve in erections at this time, compared to before surgery," with a continuous response range of 0–100%. It has been validated in men undergoing robotic-assisted RP and provides an added prognostic benefit, with a score of 0–24% being associated with a significantly greater risk of long term ED [1, 39] (Table 11.2).

Table 11.2 Questionnaires and PROs for sexual function

Questionnaire	Authors	Domains	Response options	Scoring	Target population	Administration
International Index of Erectile Function (IIEF-15)	R C Rosen et al. [34]	Erection frequency (1), erection firmness (2), penetration ability (3), maintenance frequency (4), maintenance ability (5), intercourse frequency (6), intercourse satisfaction (7), intercourse enjoyment (8), ejaculation frequency (9), orgasm frequency (10), desire frequency (11), desire level (12), overall satisfaction (13), relationship satisfaction (14), and erection confidence (15)	0–5 points Likert scale	Items scores summed Erection domain: 26 define no ED, 22–25 are categorized as mild ED, 17–21 as mild-to-moderate ED, 11–16 as moderate ED, and under 10 as severe ED	Patients with erectile dysfunction	Self-administered
International Index of Erectile Function (IIEF-5)/Sexual Health Inventory in Men (SHIM)	R C Rosen et al. [35] Alwaal A. et al. [40]	Possibility to get and maintain erection (1–4) and sexual function (2–5)	0–5 points Likert scale	Items scores summed. Total score 5–7 severe DE and 22–25 normal sexual function	Patients with erectile dysfunction	Self-administered
Male Sexual Health Questionnaire Ejaculatory Dysfunction (MSHQ EjD-Short Form)	R. C. Rosen et al. [41]	Ejaculation frequency (1), force (2), volume (3), and delay (4)	0–5 and 0–6 points Likert scale	Scoring system based on summary of items	Aging men with urogenital health concerns	Self-administered
Male Sexual Health Questionnaire (MSHQ)	R. C. Rosen et al. [36]	Erection, ejaculation, and satisfaction	0–5 and 0–6 points Likert scale	Scoring system based on summary of items	Aging men with urogenital health concerns	Self-administered
Quality of Erection Questionnaire [QEQ]	H. Porst et al. [42]	Hard enough (1), keep erection (2), time to hard enough (3), time erect (4), hardness (5), and overall quality (6)	0–5 points Likert scale	Sum of all six items is transformed onto 0–100 scale: (raw unstandardized score − 6) × 100/24	Men with erectile dysfunction	Self-administered
Erection Hardness Score/Percent Full Erection (PFE)	Mulhall et al. [38]	Single item on erection	0–5 Likert scale		Men with erectile dysfunction	Self-administered

11.4 Bowel Dysfunction

Bowel dysfunction is a possible postoperative complication after RP and it is marked by fecal incontinence (FI). FI occurs due to the loss of control of the anal sphincter. Consequently, these patients are unable to control the release of colon content, dramatically affecting self-confidence, social life, and HRQOL in general. Age is a significant predisposing factor for FI. In elderly people, FI happens in up to 4%. It is challenging to estimate the presence and the entity of bowel dysfunction before and after RP. Bishoff et al. showed a higher prevalence of less than monthly FI in men after the perineal versus retropubic approach [43]. Namiki et al. showed no significant difference in bowel complication rates in men with retropubic, perineal, or laparoscopic RP [44].

Even if this complication may appear after radical prostatectomy, it's much more common after RT and systemic therapy. During radiotherapy, bowel toxicity of any level (Radiation Therapy Oncology Group (RTOG) toxicity grade >1) was reported in 53–54% of the patients at 5 years, of which 1.5–1.9% reported a RTOG grade >3 bowel morbidity [9]. The questionnaires used to date in different published series are just instruments for abundant identification of men with post-prostatectomy alterations in bowel function. Afterward, a careful medical history, physical examination, and further laboratory examination are needed [45]. By the way, mostly General Questionnaires used for quality of life evaluation are comprehensive of items about bowel function.

11.5 General Questionnaires and Quality of Life Evaluation

Over time, the number of different general HRQoL and disease-specific HRQoL questionnaires has increased tremendously, with a recent systematic review revealing 298 different questionnaires for prostate cancer [14].

Existing HRQOL instruments that have been validated for use in prostate cancer studies are limited in evaluating contemporary prostate cancer therapies. These limitations include lack of irritative and obstructive urinary symptom assessment (complementing concurrent incontinence assessment), lack of multi-item scales for measuring function-related bother, and lack of validated, multi-item summary scores to specifically measure hormonal therapy effects and their related bother [46].

General HRQoL questionnaires assess the impact of health on an individual's everyday life without an emphasis on cancer or other disease states.

One of the first validate questionnaire is the Functional Assessment of Cancer Therapy-General (FACT-G), developed in 1993 for use in oncology clinical trials. It consists of 28 questions that operate with Likert scales (5–10 options) and uses sum scores for its scoring range. It also produces subscores for physical, functional, social, and emotional well-being. Inspired by the FACT-G, the Functional-Assessment of Cancer Therapy-Prostate (FACT-P) device was developed in 1997 and was the first HRQoL questionnaire specific to prostate cancer. FACT-P consists of 27 general questions from FACT-G along with 13 prostate cancer-specific questions and uses the same Likert scale and sum scores. In addition to general physical, emotional, and social well-being, FACT-P addresses sexual, urinary, and bowel domains. It has received high scores for content validity, internal consistency, interpretability, and responsiveness [47].

One of the most used general HRQoL questionnaire is the University of California Los Angeles Prostate Cancer Index (UCLA-PCI), collecting detailed information about bowel, sexual, and urinary function. UCLA-PCI consists of 20 questions that address impairments in sexual, urinary, and bowel domains [48]—9 sexual, 6 urinary, and 5 bowel. Each of the six disease-targeted scales was converted linearly to a 0–100 possible score range, with higher scores representing better outcomes. Of note, a condensed version of the UCLA-PCI, termed the UCLA-PCI short form (UCLA-PCI-SF), was developed in an effort to minimize the question burden of the original device [49]. Using data from the original PCI validation sample, duplicative items were eliminated while maintaining excellent reliability and validity. The Expanded Prostate Cancer Index Composite (EPIC) is a 50-question questionnaire that is an update of UCLA-PCI, with 30 additional questions on urinary and hormone function and bother scales [46], including urinary incontinence and irritation/obstruction items, along with bowel, sexual, and vitality/hormonal domains, each with function and bother subdomains. Although comprehensive, its initial 50-item version is a lengthy tool to administer and its length can be even more problematic when combined with other patient-report questionnaires.

EPIC-50 has lower construct validity and responsiveness scores than UCLA-PCI but might be more suitable for patients undergoing radiation therapy given its additional questions [50].

Although comprehensive, initial 50-item version is a lengthy tool to administer and its length can be even more problematic when combined with other patient-report questionnaires. Therefore, Szymanski et al. [50] developed a shorter version, the EPIC-26 instrument, containing 5 multi-item domains: urinary incontinence (4 items), urinary irritation/obstruction (4 items), bowel (6 items), sexual (6 items), and vitality/hormonal function (5 items); in addition, the EPIC-26 retains the single-item measure of overall urinary bother from the UCLA-PCI.

The European Organization for Research and Treatment of Cancer Quality of Life Questionnaire (EORTC QLQ-C30) contains scales and items addressing the functional aspects of HRQOL and symptoms that commonly occur in cancer patients. There are extensive reports on the validity and reliability of the QLQ-C30 used in a wide range of diagnostic and treatment settings [8]. The EORTC employs a modular approach to assessing cancer patients' HRQOL, including a core questionnaire, the QLQ-C30, a 30-question questionnaire intended for use across a wide spectrum of patient populations, and supplemental questionnaire modules, designed to assess HRQOL issues most relevant to a specific patient population.

De Nunzio et al. have recently evaluated the role of preoperative QL as a possible risk factor for post-RARP early and late urinary incontinence and the possible effect of preoperative QL on post-RARP lower urinary tract symptoms (LUTS) and ED using the EORTC-QLQ C30. Through a retrospective analysis of a prospectively maintained database of men who underwent RARP, it was seen, in line with previous experiences, that there were no clinical significant changes (less than 5 points) in the overall symptom and functional score (QLQ-30) at 6 years after surgery. It was demonstrated, in accordance to the guidelines for interpreting EORTC-QLQ-C30 scores, that a mean change in total score of more than 5 points may be considered clinically significant [51].

The EORTC-QLQ-PR25 was developed as a joint project of the EORTC Quality of Life and Genitourinary Cancer Groups in 2008, as prostate-specific HRQoL questionnaire that is consistent with the EORTC's broader measurement strategy [52].

It contains 25 Likert scale questions (4 options per question) across sexual, urinary, bowel, and hormonal domains. It is often given alongside the EORTC QLQ-Core 30; together, the two surveys provide one of the more comprehensive HRQoL assessments of all available tools.

The STAR system ("Symptom Tracking and Reporting") was initially developed for use by patients receiving outpatient chemotherapy and was found to be feasible for both clinic-based and home-based internet reporting in diverse populations, including those with no prior computer experience, lower educational levels, and high symptom burdens. STAR is a flexible interface which allows administration of questions to patients via the Web, either from clinic-based computers or from home. Data collected by STAR are exported to the electronic health record and clinical trials database for clinicians and investigators to view results.

Vickers et al. in 2010 adapted the STAR system to record data on functional recovery after radical prostatectomy. It contains six questions about the erectile function and six questions about the urinary function, two questions about bowel, and a simple 0–10 scale of global health-related quality of life to give a total of 15 questions. The validation of STAR system has obtained very high response rates, and this instrument demonstrates excellent psychometric validity (Table 11.3).

Table 11.3 Questionaries and PROs for urinary, sexual, and bowel functions

Questionnaire	Authors	Domains	Response options	Scoring	Target population	Administration
FACT-P/G (Functional Assessment of Cancer Therapy-Prostate)	Esper et al. [53]	6 domains, 39 items about QoL, physical and mental status, and urinary, sexual, and bowel dysfunctions	5-point Likert scales	Item scores are added to give summary score for each domain and a total FACT-P score Higher scores = better QoL	Men with localized or metastatic prostate cancer	Self-administered in 8–10 min
UCLA-PCI (University of California-Los Angeles Prostate Cancer Index)	Litwin et al. [54]	6 domains (20 items): Urinary function (5), sexual function (8), bowel function (4), urinary bother (1), sexual bother (1), and bowel bother (1)	3- to 5-point Likert scales	Item scores summed for the function scales and all domain scores linearly transformed to 0–100 scales. Higher scores = better QoL	Men treated for localized early-stage prostate cancer	Self-administered in 8–10 min
EPIC-26 (Expanded Prostate Index Composite-26)	Szymanski et al. [50]	4 domains (26 items): Urinary domain with incontinence subscale (4), irritation/obstruction subscale (4), overall urinary bother item (1), bowel domain (6), sexual domain (6), and vitality/hormonal domain (5)	4- and 5-point Likert scales	Item scores summed for each scale and linearly transformed to 0–100 scale. Higher scores = better QoL	Men treated for early-stage prostate cancer	Self-administered in 10 min

EPIC-50 (Expanded Prostate Index Composite)	Wei et al. [46]	4 domains (50 items): Urinary (12)—Function (5) and bother (7); bowel (14)—Function (7) and bother (7); sexual (13)—Function (9) and bother (4); hormonal (11)—Function (5) and bother (6)	3- to 5-point Likert scales	Item scores summed for each domain and linearly transformed to 0–100 scale. Higher scores = better QoL	Men treated for localized prostate cancer	Self-administered in 15–20 min
QLQ-PR25 (EORTC Prostate-Specific Module)	van Andel et al. [52]	6 domains (25 items): Urinary symptoms (8), incontinence aid (1), bowel symptoms (4), hormonal treatment-related symptoms (6), sexual active (2), and sexual functioning (4)	4-point Likert scales	Item and scale scores transformed to a 0–100 scale. Higher scores = worsening symptoms or better functioning	Men with early or advanced localized prostate cancer	Self-administered in 5–10 min
STAR (Symptom Tracking and Reporting)	Vickers et al. [13]	4 domains (15 items): Sexual function (6 items), urinary function (5 items), bowel function (2 items), and overall quality of life (1 item)	3- to 6-point Likert scales and one 11-point Likert scale	Item scores summed for the urinary and sexual function scales to give domain scores. Domain scores can also be transformed to a 0–100 scale	Men treated for early-stage prostate cancer with radical prostatectomy	Self-administered

11.6 Conclusion

In conclusion, radical prostatectomy patients experience numerous postoperative challenges such as regaining sexual, bowel, and urinary function, which can negatively impact their quality of life (QoL). Therefore, it is important for clinicians and investigators to rigorously assess QoL-related outcomes to effectively incorporate these considerations into treatment decisions. Patient-reported outcomes (PROs) are increasingly being used to assess symptoms, function, and HRQL/QoL, providing valuable data on the impact of health problems and related treatments on patients' lives. With the increasing number of general and disease-specific HRQoL questionnaires, it is essential to use the appropriate tools to measure the impact of prostate cancer treatment on patients' QoL. This chapter highlights the main questionnaires used to assess QoL in prostate cancer patients, emphasizing the importance of incorporating patient-reported outcomes in clinical decision-making.

References

1. Cooper CA, Sloan MJ, Ba AS, Fantus RJ, Raheem OA. A historical and contemporary review of questionnaires used in the management of post-radical prostatectomy patients. Sex Med Rev. 2022;10(4):681–90. https://doi.org/10.1016/j.sxmr.2022.04.003.
2. Hanson ED, Stopforth CK, Alzer M, Carver J, Lucas AR, Whang YE, et al. Body composition, physical function and quality of life in healthy men and across different stages of prostate cancer. Prostate Cancer Prostatic Dis. 2021;24(3):725–32.
3. Lardas M, Liew M, van den Bergh RC, De Santis M, Bellmunt J, Van den Broeck T, et al. Quality of life outcomes after primary treatment for clinically localised prostate cancer: a systematic review. Eur Urol. 2017;72(6):869–85.
4. Giesler RB, Miles BJ, Cowen ME, Kattan MW. Assessing quality of life in men with clinically localized prostate cancer: development of a new instrument for use in multiple settings. Qual Life Res. 2000;9(6):645–65.
5. Bourke L, Boorjian SA, Briganti A, Klotz L, Mucci L, Resnick MJ, et al. Survivorship and improving quality of life in men with prostate cancer. Eur Urol. 2015;68(3):374–83.
6. Spratt DE, Shore N, Sartor O, Rathkopf D, Olivier K. Treating the patient and not just the cancer: therapeutic burden in prostate cancer. Prostate Cancer Prostatic Dis. 2021;24(3):647–61. https://doi.org/10.1038/s41391-021-00328-1.
7. Hartmann U, Burkart M. Erectile dysfunctions in patient-physician communication: optimized strategies for addressing sexual issues and the benefit of using a patient questionnaire. J Sex Med. 2007;4(1):38–46.
8. Jiang C, Fedewa SA, Wen Y, Jemal A, Han X. Shared decision making and prostate-specific antigen based prostate cancer screening following the 2018 update of USPSTF screening guideline. Prostate Cancer Prostatic Dis. 2021;24(1):77–80. https://doi.org/10.1038/s41391-020-0227-1.
9. Mottet N, Bellmunt J, Briers E, van den Bergh RCN, Bolla M, van Casteren NJ, et al. 2023 EAU guidelines on prostate cancer. Update. 2015;53:31–45. http://www.uroweb.org/fileadmin/tx_eauguidelines/2005/Pocket/Prostate_Cancer.pdf.
10. Narang GL, Pannell SC, Laviana AA, Huen KHY, Izard J, Smith AB, et al. Patient-reported outcome measures in urology. Curr Opin Urol. 2017;27(4):366–74.
11. Kim JS, Taaffe DR, Galvão DA, Hart NH, Gray E, Ryan CJ, et al. Exercise in advanced prostate cancer elevates myokine levels and suppresses in-vitro cell growth. Prostate Cancer Prostatic Dis. 2022;25(1):86–92.

12. Protopapa E, van der Meulen J, Moore CM, Smith SC. Patient-reported outcome (PRO) questionnaires for men who have radical surgery for prostate cancer: a conceptual review of existing instruments. BJU Int. 2017;120(4):468–81.
13. Vickers AJ, Savage CJ, Shouery M, Eastham JA, Scardino PT, Basch EM. Validation study of a web-based assessment of functional recovery after radical prostatectomy. Health Qual Life Outcomes. 2010;8:82.
14. Hamoen EHJ, De Rooij M, Witjes JA, Barentsz JO, Rovers MM. Measuring health-related quality of life in men with prostate cancer: a systematic review of the most used questionnaires and their validity. Urol Oncol Semin Orig Investig. 2015;33(2):69.e19–28.
15. Lepor H, Kaci L, Xue X. Continence following radical retropubic prostatectomy using self-reporting instruments. J Urol. 2004;171(3):1212–5.
16. Cestari A, Rigatti L, Lughezzani G, Guazzoni G. How should we report incontinence after radical prostatectomy? J Urol. 2010;184(3):829–30.
17. Schumacher FA, Helenowski IB, Sun Z, Oswald LB, Gonzalez BD, Moses KA, et al. Treatment decision-making among patients with metastatic prostate cancer: impact of decision locus of control on functional outcomes and decision satisfaction. Prostate Cancer Prostatic Dis. 2023;26(1):201–6.
18. Wei JT, Dunn RL, Marcovich R, Montie JE, Sanda MG. Prospective assessment of patient reported urinary continence after radical prostatectomy. J Urol. 2000;164(3 Pt 1):744–8.
19. Kadono Y, Ueno S, Iwamoto D, Takezawa Y, Nohara T, Izumi K, et al. Chronological urodynamic evaluation of changing bladder and urethral functions after robot-assisted radical prostatectomy. Urology. 2015;85(6):1441–7.
20. Sandhu JS, Breyer B, Comiter C, Eastham JA, Gomez C, Kirages DJ, et al. Incontinence after prostate treatment: AUA/SUFU guideline. J Urol. 2019;202(2):369–78.
21. Barry MJ, Fowler FJ, O'Leary MP, Bruskewitz RC, Holtgrewe HL, Mebust WK, et al. The American Urological Association symptom index for benign prostatic hyperplasia. J Urol. 1992;148(5):1549–57.
22. Lerner LB, McVary KT, Barry MJ, Bixler BR, Dahm P, Das AK, et al. Management of lower urinary tract symptoms attributed to benign prostatic hyperplasia: AUA guideline part I—initial work-up and medical management. J Urol. 2021;206(4):806–17.
23. Griffith JW. Self-report measurement of lower urinary tract symptoms: a commentary on the literature since 2011. Curr Urol Rep. 2012;13(6):420–6.
24. Bayoud Y, de la Taille A, Ouzzane A, Ploussard G, Allory Y, Yiou R, et al. International Prostate Symptom Score is a predictive factor of lower urinary tract symptoms after radical prostatectomy. Int J Urol. 2015;22(3):283–7.
25. Leyh-Bannurah SR, Wagner C, Schuette A, Liakos N, Karagiotis T, Mendrek M, et al. Improvement of quality of life and symptom burden after robot-assisted radical prostatectomy in patients with moderate to severe LUTS. Sci Rep. 2021;11(1):16757.
26. Walker NF, Canagasingham A, Van Diepen D, Pirpiris A, Tse V, Leslie S, et al. Lower urinary tract functional assessment of men undergoing radical prostatectomy: correlation of preoperative clinical and urodynamic parameters. Int Neurourol J. 2021;25(2):157–63.
27. Fayers PM, Machin D. Quality of life: the assessment, analysis and interpretation of patient-reported outcomes. 2nd ed. Chichester: Wiley; 2007.
28. Wein AJ. ICIQ: a brief and robust measure for evaluating the symptoms and impact of urinary incontinence. J Urol. 2005;173(3):908–9.
29. Machioka K, Kadono Y, Naito R, Nakashima K, Iijima M, Kawaguchi S, et al. Evaluating urinary incontinence before and after radical prostatectomy using the International Consultation on Incontinence Questionnaire-Short Form. Neurourol Urodyn. 2019;38(2):726–33.
30. Abrams P, Avery K, Gardener N, Donovan J. The International Consultation on Incontinence Modular Questionnaire: www.iciq.net. J Urol. 2006;175(3 Pt 1):1063–6.
31. Suskind AM, Dunn RL, Morgan DM, Delancey JOL, McGuire EJ, Wei JT. The Michigan Incontinence Symptom Index (M-ISI): a clinical measure for type, severity, and bother related to urinary incontinence. Neurourol Urodyn. 2014;33(7):1128–34.

32. Helgason ÁR, Adolfsson J, Dickman P, Fredrikson M, Arver S, Steineck G. Waning sexual function—the most important disease-specific distress for patients with prostate cancer. Br J Cancer. 1996;73(11):1417–21.
33. Liatsikos EN, Assimakopoulos K, Stolzenburg JU. Quality of life after radical prostatectomy. Urol In. 2008;80(3):226–30.
34. Rosen RC, Riley A, Wagner G, Osterloh IH, Kirkpatrick J, Mishra A. The International Index of Erectile Function (IIEF): a multidimensional scale for assessment of erectile dysfunction. Urology. 1997;49(6):822–30.
35. Rosen RC, Cappelleri JC, Smith MD, Lipsky J, Peñ BM. Development and evaluation of an abridged, 5-item version of the International Index of Erectile Function (IIEF-5) as a diagnostic tool for erectile dysfunction. Int J Impot Res. 1999;11(6):319–26.
36. Rosen RC, Catania J, Pollack L, Althof S, O'Leary M, Seftel AD. Male Sexual Health Questionnaire (MSHQ): scale development and psychometric validation. Urology. 2004;64(4):777–82.
37. Yafi FA, Huynh LM, Ahlering T, Rosen R. What is a "Validated Questionnaire"? A critical review of erectile function assessment. J Sex Med. 2020;17(5):849–60.
38. Mulhall JP, Goldstein I, Bushmakin AG, Cappelleri JC, Hvidsten K. Validation of the erection hardness score. J Sex Med. 2007;4(6):1626–34.
39. Huynh LM, Osann K, Skarecky D, Ahlering TE. Predictive modelling of 2-year potency outcomes using a novel 90-day erection fullness scale after robot-assisted radical prostatectomy. BJU Int. 2018;122(2):249–54.
40. Alwaal A, Awad M, Boggs N, Kuzbel J, Snoad B. Sexual Health Inventory for Men Questionnaire as a screening method for erectile dysfunction in a general urology clinic. Sex Med. 2020;8(4):660–3.
41. Rosen RC, Catania JA, Althof SE, Pollack LM, O'Leary M, Seftel AD, et al. Development and validation of four-item version of Male Sexual Health Questionnaire to assess ejaculatory dysfunction. Urology. 2007;69(5):805–9.
42. Porst H, Gilbert C, Collins S, Huang X, Symonds T, Stecher V, et al. Development and validation of the quality of erection questionnaire. J Sex Med. 2007;4(2):372–81.
43. Bishoff JT, Motley G, Optenberg SA, Stein CR, Moon KA, Browning SM, et al. Incidence of fecal and urinary incontinence following radical perineal and retropubic prostatectomy in a national population. J Urol. 1998;160(2):454–8.
44. Namiki S, Egawa S, Terachi T, Matsubara A, Igawa M, Terai A, et al. Changes in quality of life in first year after radical prostatectomy by retropubic, laparoscopic, and perineal approach: multi-institutional longitudinal study in Japan. Urology. 2006;67(2):321–7.
45. Kirschner-Hermanns R, Jakse G. Quality of life following radical prostatectomy. Crit Rev Oncol Hematol. 2002;43(2):141–51.
46. Wei JT, Dunn RL, Litwin MS, Sandler HM, Sanda MG. Development and validation of the Expanded Prostate Cancer Index Composite (EPIC) for comprehensive assessment of health-related quality of life in men with prostate cancer. Urology. 2000;56(6):899–905.
47. Cella DF, Tulsky DS, Gray G, Sarafian B, Linn E, Bonomi A, et al. The functional assessment of cancer therapy scale: development and validation of the general measure. J Clin Oncol. 1993;11(3):570–9.
48. Litwin MS, Hays RD, Fink A, Ganz PA, Leake B, Brook RH. The UCLA Prostate Cancer Index: development, reliability, and validity of a health-related quality of life measure. Med Care. 1998;36(7):1002–12. https://doi.org/10.1097/00005650-199807000-00007. PMID: 9674618.
49. Litwin MS, McGuigan KA. Accuracy of recall in health-related quality-of-life assessment among men treated for prostate cancer. J Clin Oncol. 1999;17(9):2882–8.
50. Szymanski KM, Wei JT, Dunn RL, Sanda MG. Development and validation of an abbreviated version of the expanded prostate cancer index composite instrument for measuring health-related quality of life among prostate cancer survivors. Urology. 2010;76(5):1245–50.

51. De Nunzio C, Pastore AL, Lombardo R, Cancrini F, Carbone A, Fuschi A, et al. The EORTC quality of life questionnaire predicts early and long-term incontinence in patients treated with robotic assisted radical prostatectomy: analysis of a large single center cohort. Urol Oncol Semin Orig Investig. 2019;37(12):1006–13. https://doi.org/10.1016/j.urolonc.2019.06.024.
52. van Andel G, Bottomley A, Fosså SD, Efficace F, Coens C, Guerif S, et al. An international field study of the EORTC QLQ-PR25: a questionnaire for assessing the health-related quality of life of patients with prostate cancer. Eur J Cancer. 2008;44(16):2418–24.
53. Esper P, Mo F, Chodak G, Sinner M, Cella D, Pienta KJ. Measuring quality of life in men with prostate cancer using the functional assessment of cancer therapy-prostate instrument. Urology. 1997;50(6):920–8.
54. Litwin MS, Hays RD, Fink A, Ganz PA, Leake B, Brook RH. The UCLA Prostate Cancer Index: development, reliability, and validity of a health-related quality of life measure. Med Care. 1998;36(7):1002–12.

MIX
Papier aus verantwortungsvollen Quellen
Paper from responsible sources
FSC® C105338

If you have any concerns about our products,
you can contact us on
ProductSafety@springernature.com

In case Publisher is established outside the EU,
the EU authorized representative is:
Springer Nature Customer Service Center GmbH
Europaplatz 3, 69115 Heidelberg, Germany

Printed by Libri Plureos GmbH
in Hamburg, Germany